FINALLY!

...A book that reveals a realistic approach to weight loss. Thank you, Stephen! *Lose Weight with The Power of One* is great and the way it reads is fabulous. After just the first few strategies I found myself thinking of them and implementing them into my own life as though they were second nature. What a powerful book. Everyone, not just the overweight, will relate to your strategies and realistically apply them to their lives. All will benefit from them and live with them. *Lose Weight with The Power of One* will be a mandatory read for all my clients.

Melinda M. Brenner, ATC, CSCS
Certified Fitness Specialist, Athletic Trainer, and Strength Coach

I'm excited about *Lose Weight with The Power of One*. After the first page I couldn't put it down!! Finally, a book that explains a process of living a healthy lifestyle without pushing any fad diet or strict guidelines. As I read *Lose Weight with The Power of One*, I constantly thought of how my clients were experiencing the same thoughts and feelings, and going through the same trials and tribulations as the characters. This book explains the basic concepts that will help *anyone* improve their life or lose weight. I will be using *Lose Weight with The Power of One* with all of my clients, and as a source of encouragement for myself.

Dr. Patrick S. Hagerman, Ed.D., CSCS*D, NSCA-CPT*D, USAW,
ACSM University of Tulsa, Dept. of Athletic Tr~~~~ **rcise**
& Sport Science; President, Quest Per~~~~
2002 NSCA Personal Train~~~~

I am excited to be able to recommend this book to my clients! Stephen has put together a brilliant real-life example of what I teach on a daily basis. He has shown that it is possible to make life-changing, long-term, healthy behavior changes that make excess weight melt off. He has given us a wonderful way of prioritizing life, food, and one's relationship to both. Thank you for this book.

Amy Burris Burrow, BS, RD, LD
Registered, Licensed Dietitian; Owner, Gentle Nutrition Consulting Services; Provider of Medical Nutrition Therapy, Killeen Texas

Excellent! *Lose Weight with The Power of One's* eight strategies are right on target. I especially *love* the fact that the book's goal is "to gain health" and not only lose weight. This book is great. I will recommend it to my friends and clients.

Sandy Guess Couvillon, MS, LDN, RD
Author of The Idiot's Guide to Weight Loss, part of the Orange series of Complete Idiot Guide books

Lose Weight with The Power of One has Oprah written all over it!

Regina Sara Ryan, Co-author with Dr. John Travis, Wellness Workbook, as well as Simply Well: Choices for a Healthier Life, and After Surgery, Illness and Trauma: 10 Steps to Renewed Energy.

I loved *Lose Weight with The Power of One!* Using fictional characters is a wonderful way to increase understanding of the difficult trials of weight management. The principles of *Lose Weight with The Power of One* are simple, sensible, and effective. Not only will I recommend this book to my clients, I have begun to use its strategies myself! My hope is that *Lose Weight with The Power of One* will help revolutionize America's obsession with quick weight-loss gimmicks, and help put an end to diet quackery. Many blessings to Stephen Moss!!

Karen C. Godette, MS, RD
Nu-Abundance Nutrition Consulting Services, Chesapeake, Virginia

Stephen Moss has *nailed* the whole issue of healthy eating! While reading *Lose Weight with The Power of One* it really felt as though he and I had been talking for years, and that he has listened to every consultation I ever gave to a client. Truly amazing and heartwarming! This book is simultaneously basic and wondrous! A true "return to nutritional sanity." Not only an avid read, but profoundly needed.

Denia Mette', CN M.ED, CN, DD
Degrees in Counseling, Nutrition and Theology

Congratulations, Stephen Moss! I recommend *Lose Weight with The Power of One* to anyone who wants to lose weight and doesn't know where to start — or to someone who has tried in the past and failed. This is not another "how to" book, but a "how you can!" Through some powerful scenes, Stephen Moss has created visuals that will long be with us, showing us that the future is all about healthy lifestyle choices.

Brenda L. Marshall, B.Sc., R.Dt.
President, CQI Consulting (Continuous Quality Improvements)

Lose Weight with The Power of One is a novel way to portray the challenges and solutions to weight-loss/control. Several times I was brought to tears by the struggles of the characters Janice and Karen. On a factual level this book rightfully avoids the pitfalls of all the other books out there, by avoiding the pseudoscientific explanations of macro and micro nutrients, etc. It offers the hows, not whys, and that's what people want and need. Oprah will love having Stephen Moss on!

Dr. Irv Rubenstein, Exercise Physiologist, President of S.T.E.P.S, Inc.

Lose Weight with The Power of One's message is simple and insightful, a winning combination!

Mary Delasantos, Certified Nutritionist
Author of She's Vegetarian – He's Not (And Living to Tell About It)

Lose Weight with The Power of One is hard to put down! Though I read as much as I can on nutrition, this is the first time I've read a weight-loss book that was entertaining. Even exciting! The amazing thing is that Stephen Moss wrote many of the same things I preach all the time — and put it in such a simple, easy-to-understand manner. I cannot think of one of my clients, much less anyone on this planet, who could not benefit from this book! I strongly recommend it.

I loved it!!! Finally a book on nutrition that gives good, sound, healthy advice! I've been looking for a way to explain how to adopt healthier eating habits without making it sound complicated and I've found it in *Lose Weight with The Power of One*. What a great book! Not only does Stephen give sound nutritional information, but he presents it in a way that's fun to read and easy to understand. I simply couldn't put the book down.

What a pleasant surprise *Lose Weight with The Power of One* was! I was expecting to review a boring weight-loss book and instead found myself immersed in an inspirational story of how a woman regains control of her body and her life! *Lose Weight with The Power of One* is so much more than a book on weight loss — it's a creative mix of storyline and valuable, usable strategies for weight loss or any other lifestyle change. I will definitely recommend this book to my students and my clients. Thank you, Stephen, for sharing your knowledge in such an entertaining way!

I truly enjoyed *Lose Weight with The Power of One*! I laughed. I cried. I felt the excitement and courage it conveyed. It's wonderful! A great way to get across the true message of how to lose weight and lead a healthy lifestyle. This outstanding novel will give courage and hope to millions of former dieters and pave the way for the nation.

Martha Gottlieb, Certified Nutritionist, Personal Trainer,
and Author of Spriggles Motivational Books for Children

I just have one word for *Lose Weight with The Power of One*—fantastic! In my years as a personal trainer I have seen many people struggle with losing weight and changing their eating habits, and I've always looked for a tool or method that would help simplify the process. And now I've found it! *Lose Weight with The Power of One* will be required reading for all my clients.

Doug Murphy, Fitness Training and Consulting, Washington D.C.
www.dougmurphy.com

I can't wait to recommend this book to my clients. What a wonderful integration of healthy lifestyle with wholesome principles. My counseling with clients utilizes each of them. I am recommending it to all my clients for weight control/healthy lifestyle. It is also how I manage my own weight.

Pat Compton, RD, LD, Consultant Dietitian
President/Owner, The Nutrition Exchange

Lose Weight with The Power of One is not only a lifestyle-changing book, it is the education I have been trying to teach my clients for over twenty years. The book applies not only to those trying to control their weight, it applies to *everyone* seeking a healthier lifestyle. I enjoyed reading it and will recommend it to all of my clients—I am keeping a copy for their reference on my shelf!

Carrie Morrow, MBA, JD
Legal-Fitness Consultant; Owner, Fitness Dynamics Training Studio,
McMurray, Pennsylvania

In a society that is at epidemic levels of obesity and overweight in adults and children, this book and philosophy is going to save lives. While creating a unique approach to capturing the audience's attention with a riveting story, Stephen Moss will change people's lives by inspiring them to develop a healthy lifestyle with this fantastic book and journey.

> *James B. Jefferson MES, C.N Exercise Physiologist; Internet Personal Trainer of the Year 1999, 2000, 2001; 18 years of experience; President, Your Personal Trainer TV. www.JamesYourPersonalTrainer.com*

I just finished reading *Lose Weight with The Power of One*. I'm so excited I can't wait to share it! I have been preaching this stuff to deaf ears for so long that I can't describe in words how thrilled I was to read in black and white the same principles I personally use and teach. We are at war with food manufacturers and advertisers every day. Thank you, Stephen, for putting it in those terms. Your book renewed my commitment as a soldier for nutritional sanity.

> *Carla J. Nichols, BS, CSCS, NSCA-CPT Certified USA Weightlifting Club Coach; Owner, Competitive Edge Personal Training, Wichita Falls, Texas*

Lose Weight with The Power of One is hard to put down! I really enjoyed reading it, and feel it has much to offer people who view changing their lifestyles a hopeless undertaking. I'm glad the book shows failure and difficulty in learning to follow a different type of plan from the typical diets. Change is never easy, and the book highlights some important points that are sure to hit home with many people. I'm looking forward to recommending it as one of my preferred references!

> *Lynn Grieger, RD, CDE Consulting Nutritionist and Freelance Author, Southwestern Vermont, specializing in diabetes, weight control, and women's issues*

Excellent!! Stephen Moss' book *Lose Weight with The Power of One* is *hope* for all. He offers commonsense approaches. This is the first book I have ever read that illustrates how weight loss can fit one's life without it being a struggle. A must read *before* considering any weight-loss program.

Rita Batheja, MS, RD, Nutritionist in private practice, Long Island, New York; Founder, Indian American Dietetic Association

Read *Lose Weight with The Power of One* with a pencil; underline and take notes because you will want to refer to it again and again. This book is a novel idea for eating well for a lifetime. It's presented in everyday language and situations, with very easy-to-understand concepts. I will recommend it to all my clients who want to improve their eating habits.

Glenn Johnson, Certified Personal Fitness Trainer;
Founder, Motion Works Fitness.

Lose Weight with The Power of One makes great use of the art of storytelling to deliver an important message for today—you can change your life! For anyone struggling with the issue of weightloss, the story stays with you like a supportive mentor and friend—encouraging and guiding you all the way to success.

Mary Ann Copson, Professional Coach, Consultant, and Certified Nutritionist, CEO, Evenstar – Peak Performance Living and Personal Growth Enhancement

Lose Weight with The Power of One is a wonderful weight-loss guide written in the form of a novel. Through the characters of Karen, Fowler, and Janice, the book clearly shows how overweight people can overcome all obstacles and win, long-term, the battle against obesity. *Lose Weight with The Power of One should be read by everyone!*

Melissa Hon-Tulchinsky, MSRD, CNSD
Clinical Dietitian and Private Nutrition Consultant

Lose Weight with The Power of One is an important new approach to weightloss! Everyone should read this accurate yet simple solution to being overweight. *Lose Weight with The Power of One* provides the diet-confused world the information it needs to face each day with a positive attitude, and to expect real results through a commonsense approach to eating.

Michael Lambeth, BS, USMA CSCS NSCA Certified Fitness Trainer, Lifestyle & Weight Management Consultant, Owner, Personalized Fitness & Nutrition, Charlotte, North Carolina

In my work with young people with disabilities I am always on the lookout for role models for them. I have found just that in a place I least expected — *Lose Weight with The Power of One*. Janice is not perfect nor is she free from fears that affect us all. As a result, she makes a perfect role model for disabled youth. Why? Because she learns from what she teaches others and struggles to apply these lessons in her own life. Role models needn't be perfect, they just need to be like Janice — kind, bright, and willing to do their best. Thank you, Stephen Moss, for giving us this gift of *Lose Weight with The Power of One*.

Dr. Linda Marie Stein, PhD, MFT.
www.disabilitycentral.com

Lose Weight with The Power of One is really the power for *all*. It's like the story of Dorothy in *The Wizard of Oz*. She had the power all along but just didn't know it. We too have the power to change our lives — and Stephen Moss shows us how to do this. How to tap into that inner strength we all have within us. I also applaud his nutrition savvy and practicality. This book is sensitively written, but most of all, powerful!

Claudia Del Vecchio, BS, CDN, CPT New York State Certified Dietitian/Nutritionist; ACE Certified Personal Trainer; Owner, Original Well-Bean Coffee Co., Inc.; Co-author, Every Which Way With Coffee

Fast-food joints read and weep! This book will be a best-seller, and what a way to fight back. Stephen has empowered the American people with *knowledge* about why we are fat and how to take control, in a touching story format. I enjoyed the word pictures throughout the book describing Fowler's home, Janice and Karen, and Courage. I look forward to seeing this book on the best-seller list and I will definitely recommend it and use it with my clients.

Della J. Bossart, Wellness Consultants, US Air Force Academy

As a personal trainer, one of the most difficult objectives is trying to identify why clients can't make changes in their nutritional habits. This book does more than just identify the problem — it expresses it in a way that thousands of people will relate to it. I have read *a lot* of diet books, but none more intriguing than *Lose Weight with The Power of One*. It's a phenomenal breakthrough in the world of proper nutrition.

Michael Villa, Certified Personal Trainer, Austin, Texas.
www.michaelvilla.com

Congrats, Stephen on a great book that helps guide people in taking their first steps toward good health and nutrition. It's refreshing in this complex world of "diets" to get back to the basics of simple, good nutrition.

Chef Stephanie Green, RD, Culinary Educator;
President, Nutrition Studio

I read *Lose Weight with The Power of One* in just part of an afternoon. This was an easy read and a step in the right direction for people who just aren't sure what to do "next" about their bodies. The approach is both clever and entertaining. It will find favor in the eyes of personal training agencies as it meets their guidelines. It will also appeal to housewives in droves. Stephen Moss is on to something!

Don Lemmon, www.aboutdiet.com

It's great! Excellent approach. *Lose Weight with The Power of One* keeps the reader involved and really changes their view on diets. What's best is that without them realizing it, the knowledge they gain from reading this book actually makes a change in their lives! *Lose Weight with The Power of One* doesn't cram a diet down your throat, but because of the information presented as a novel, teaches lifestyle changes—which ultimately is the key to success.

Dr. Sal A. Arria
CEO & CoFounder: International Sports Sciences Association

Good job! *Lose Weight with The Power of One* does not focus on weight loss, but lifestyle change. Describing simple, baby steps, Stephen Moss shows everyone how to make easy life changes that will improve their health and help them achieve their natural weight. He shows us how *planning to succeed* rather than just *planning to try* is the key to success! I urge everyone who does not believe they can get a handle on their health and weight to read *Lose Weight with The Power of One!*

Carol G. Fenwick, MHS, RD, LDN Certified Health/Fitness
Instructor, ACSM; Owner, Lifestyle Enhancement Center

I thoroughly enjoyed *Lose Weight with The Power of One*. The book is as entertaining as it is educational. Fowler, Janice, and Karen's experience changing their lifestyle is *inspirational*. As a Registered Dietitian who specializes in behavior changes and not diets, this is very refreshing. I will definitely recommend this book to all my clients!

Diane Machcinski, M.Ed., RD Director, A+ Nutrition specializing in weight management, diabetes, and cardiac clients; 2000 California Dietetic Association's award winner for Excellence in Private Practice, Business and Communications

Editor's note: *We regret that due to the overwhelming number of endorsements the pre-publication edition of Lose Weight with The Power of One received, most, due to space constraints, could not be included in the book.*

Lose Weight with
THE POWER
OF ONE

A MOTIVATIONAL JOURNEY
TO NUTRITIONAL SANITY

Stephen Moss

Project coordinator:
Chaz Consultants

First edition August 2003

Published by Stephen Moss

P.O. Box 68
Postal Station Victoria
Westmount Qc Canada
H3Z 2V4

Printed in Canada

ISBN: 0-9733228-0-2

For Natalia,

my first priority

Table of Contents

ACKNOWLEDGMENTS

No book, especially one that breaks new ground in the complex field of weight loss, can be created alone. Behind the name on the cover are many dedicated professionals whose efforts combined to produce this labor of love.

I want to first thank the two people who inadvertently started me on this journey. Maria Odivic, for calling and asking me to help get her nutritional life under control, and Wilma Magonet, weight-loss counselor, who read a copy of the strategies I created for Maria, and said those fateful words: "You should put this into a book."

I also need to acknowledge the hundreds of researchers in the weight-loss field whose work I freely drew on. Though outshone by the "fad diet camp," they hold the true answer to permanent weight control.

As well, my sincere appreciation goes out to the over 100 professionals from across North America who read my manuscript and offered their suggestions and enthusiastic support. As each of those letters came in, my spirits soared. These physicians, dietitians, nutritionists, and fitness specialists embraced my vision and approach, and truly became a part of *The Power of One* family. Their names are listed on the following pages.

Special mention needs to be given to Dr. Rudy Brenner MD, CCFP, Dr. Sal Arria, and Lynn Grieger, RD, CDE, for their early support. As well as Dr. Irv Rubenstein and Dr. Patrick S. Hagerman for their attention to detail.

I also want to thank Dr. Linda Marie Stein for reading my manuscript from the point of view of the physically disabled. Her contribution helped me to better portray the character of Janice — making her an inspiration for everyone.

Finally, I want to thank all those, professional and laypeople alike, who have written to say how *Lose Weight with The Power of One* touched their lives and the lives of family members and clients, helping each begin their journey toward greater health and permanent weight loss.

IN ALPHABETICAL ORDER, *I wish to thank:*

Christopher Aiello, *CFT, Milwaukee,* WI

Dr. Sal A. Arria, *CEO & CoFounder, International Sports Sciences Association,* CA

Alice Baland, *MA, LPC, RD/LD,* Plano, TX

Rita Batheja, *MS, RD, CDN,* Baldwin, NY

Barbara Beznos, *RD, LD/N,* Farmington Hills, MI

Dan Bialik *CFI,* Overland, MO

Della J. Bossart, *Wellness Consultant,* Colorado Springs, CO

Fitzroy Bramble, *Pro-bodybuilder and NFPT, FRA, AFAA,* Malden, MA

Melinda M. Brenner, *ATC, CSCS,* Long Branch, NJ

Dr. Rudy Brenner, *MD, CCFP,* Montreal, Canada

Amy Burris-Burrow, *RD, LD,* Salado, TX

David Calvert, *BA, CSCS,* Tucson, AZ

Andrea Chernus *MS, RD,* New York, NY

Frank Claps, Hellertown, PA

Pat Compton, *RD, LD,* Sterling, VA

Mary Ann Copson, *CN,* Shipman, VA

Sandy Guess Couvillon, *MS, LDN, RD,* Alexandria, LA

Barbara Cox, *RD,* Reno, NV

Terri Crosby-Hornbaker, *CH, CN,* Boulder, CO

Kathleen D'Achille Kintzle, *PHarmD, MEd,* Greenville, SC

David J. DeHart, *BS, CN,* Marcellus, MI

Mary Delasantos, *CN,* Castle Rock, CO

Claudia Del Vecchio, *BS, CDN, CPT,* Webster, NY

Natalie Dickstein, *RD, Certified Diabetes Educator,* Poughkeepsie, NY

Anne Dubner, *RD, LD,* Houston, TX

Lynda Binius Enright, *MS, RD, LD,* St. Louis Park, MN

Carol Fenwick, *MHS, RD, LDN,* Arden, NC

Nancy Ferriello, *MS, RD, CD-N,* Westport, CT

C. Allen Figg, *MS, CSCS, RCEP,* Santa Fe, NM

Kathryn Fink, *RD, LD,* Irving, TX

Carol-lee Fisher, *CNE,* San Antonio, TX

Jan Fortina, *RD, LD,* Indian Head Park, IL
Sally Gabriel, *MA, MBA, CN,* Sarasota, FL
Marjorie Geiser, *RD, NSCA-CPT,* Running Springs, CA
Sheila Ginsberg, *MS, RD, CDE,* Avila Beach, CA
Karen C. Godette, *MS, RD,* Chesapeake, VA
P.M. Goodman, *DDS, MSc, PhD,* Kettering, OH
Christine Goodson, *RD, LD,* Houston, TX
Martha Gottlieb, *Certified Nutritionist, Personal Trainer,* Harbor
  Springs, MI
Chef Stephanie Green, *RD, Culinary Educator,* Phoenix, AZ
Lynn Grieger, *RD, CDE,* Arlington, VT
Dr. Patrick S. Hagerman, *EdD, CSCS*D, NSCA-CPT*D, USAW,
  ACSM,* Nowata, OK
Patricia Henry, *MEd, RD, LD, CDE*, Tomball, TX
Lynn Hinderliter, *CN, LNC,* Macomb, IL
Melissa Hon-Tulchinsky, *MSRD, CNSD,* Greenville, DE
Dale Huff, *RD, CSCS,* St. Louis, MO
Ann Hunter, *PhD, RD, LD, FADA,* Wichita, KS
Michael Iserman, *CSCS,* Brooklyn Park, MN
James B. Jefferson, *MES, CN, Exercise Physiologist,* Medford, NJ
Derek Johnson, *Personal Dietitian,* Los Angeles, CA
Glenn Johnson, *CFT,* Torrance, CA
Gina E. Kennedy, *CN,* Skaneateles, NY
Sylvie L. Kessem, *Naturopathy Student,* Monteal, Canada
Don Lemmon, *aboutdiet.com,* Las Vegas, NV
Michael Lambeth, *BS, USMA, CSCS, CPT,* Mathews, NC
Joan Levinthal, *RD,* Woodland Hills, CA
Diane Machcinski, *MEd, RD,* San Diego, CA
Wilma Magonet, Montreal, Canada
Don Mankie, *RD,* Salem, VA
Dr. Patti Mantia, *EdD, CSCS, HFI,* Mansfield, MA
Paul Marino, *PT, OCS, CSCS, CPT-NSCA,* Marietta, GA
Brenda L. Marshall, *BSc, RDt,* St. John's, Canada
Lee McDonagh, *RD, CDE,* Canton, MI
Maryann Meade, *MS, RD, CD-N,* Wallingford, CT

Denia Mette', *MED, CN, DD,* Las Vegas, NV

Laurie Meyer, *MS, RD, CD,* Grafton, WI

Carrie Morrow, *MBA, JD,* McMurray, PA

Doug Murphy, *CPT,* Miami, FL

Bonnie Murphy, *PFT,* Anchorage, AK

Nina Myers, B.Ed.(Phys.Ed.) *Trainer of fitness instructors,* Montreal, Canada

Judy Nicassio, *CN,* Hoffman Estates, IL

Carla J. Nichols, *CSCS,* Wichita Falls, TX

Diana Pace, *GM,* Highland Village, TX

Natasha Patton, *RD, RN,* Surrey, Canada

Susan Perry, *BS, CPT,* Austin, TX

Clint Phillips, *ACE CFT, LWMC, CES, NSCA, CSCS,* Evanston, IL

Marcia Poe, *RDH, MS,* Belton, MO

Robert Raymond, *President, RR Personal Training Inc.,* Littleton CO

Jeanie Redick, *CN,* Roanoke, VA

Gay Riley, *MS, RD, LD,* Richardson, TX

Sue Roselle, *MS, CN,* Fairfax, VA.

Dr. Irv Rubenstein, Nashville, TN

Regina Sara Ryan, *Author, Editor, Hohm Press,* Prescott AZ

Kerry Seymour, *MS, RD, CDE,* Reno, NV

David Sloniegura *PFT,* Albany, NY

Sarah Krumme Stahr, *MS, CPT, CSCS,* Cincinnati, OH

Linda Marie Stein, *PhD, MFT,* Long Beach, CA

Lisa Smiley, *CSCS, NSCA-CPT*,* Cannon Falls, MN

Andrea Smith, *MSc, RD,* Calgary, Canada

Lisa Spallitta, *CPT,* Baltimore, MD

Paul Stofko, *BS, CSCS,* Chesterton, IN

Jackie Storm, *PhD, CNS,* Forest City, PA

Arlene Swantko, *RD, LD,* Columbia, MD

Audean Tuell, *Certified Nutritionist,* Bedford, TX

Michael Villa, *CPT,* Austin, TX

Vadim Vilensky, *MS, CSCS,* Scarsdale, NY

Kristin White, *Master Fitness by Phone Coach,* Alpharetta, GA

FOREWORD

Like many physicians, my time is limited. So when Stephen Moss asked me to read *Lose Weight with The Power of One*, I hesitated. He then said, "Just start it, read a page or two, and if it's not for you, that's okay." Under these conditions I agreed. After the first few pages, however, I found that I couldn't put the book down, and read it in its entirety in a single day.

Stephen Moss has taken the latest in nutritional research, reworded it into plain English, and presented it in a way that is not only highly motivational, but exciting!

This is not a diet book. It is a well-thought-out blueprint for permanently changing one's nutritional life. By simplifying the weight-loss process into eight easy strategies based on commonsense and real life, *Lose Weight with The Power of One* has the potential to change the lives of those millions who have dieted and failed, and now view weightloss as hopeless.

Lose Weight with The Power of One emphasizes personalizing a plan to fit individual needs, empowering each of us to take control of our own choices, and to take small, doable steps toward the goal of better nutritional health. These are important messages that need to be heard and understood.

Lose Weight with The Power of One also eliminates the need to count fat grams, calories, or anything else. Instead, by the end of the book, the reader, almost without being aware of it, will have internalized a new and healthier way of eating.

And this is the only true answer to permanent weight loss.

I encourage everyone to read this book thoroughly, and then read it again. It will change your life.

Rudy Brenner, MD, CCFP

AUTHOR'S PREFACE

I grew up in a household where my parents and sister were overweight. But I was one of those irritating types who could eat as they please and never gain an ounce—until I turned thirty.

Then it hit me too.

Overnight it seemed my weight jumped up thirty pounds. I "crash-dieted" that weight off, patted myself on the back, then turned around and gained it back plus a little more. This became my pattern for years —and I tried them all. Low-fat diets, low-calorie diets, protein diets and "last as long as you can" starvation diets!

I looked to the so-called experts for help. And all I found was confusion. One camp said the road to weightloss began with high protein and high fat. The other swore it was low fat and high carbohydrates. Yet others told me it had to do with sugar and insulin and even my blood type.

It made me crazy! Do I really have to follow someone else's nutritional lifestyle, I wondered. One that doesn't fit me at all? One that I already knew from experience would inevitably lead to anxiety, frustration, guilt, and that overwhelming sense of failure each time I ate what I really craved.

To make sense of it I began to read everything I could find on weightloss, and during the next ten years became a Specialist in Weight Management, a Lifestyle and Weight Management Consultant, and a Certified Fitness Trainer. What I was mostly, though, was someone on a journey to find a solution to the question: How could I lose weight easily, and keep it off, without having *any* diet interfere with my life?

What I discovered during those ten years was that the answer was there all along, hidden beneath the mountains of quick-fix fad diets. Written by dozens of well-meaning professionals, it had been proven over decades, and endorsed by every major medical and nutritional association. But the answer was so buried within reams of dry clinical studies that it had to be mined, brought out bit by bit as I uncovered a nugget of understanding here, a seam of truth there.

As I suspected, the answer did not lie within any particular camp. The solution to permanent weightloss turned out to be embedded in commonsense and real life. It also took into account everyone's personal tastes and urges and bad days.

I gradually applied what I discovered, and began to lose weight—slowly, continuously, and *easily*. *Without dieting*. Until I lost all I had to. And for the past five years I've lived life as someone thin, fit, and healthy. I'd found the answer for my wife and myself, and we went on happily with our lives.

The story might well have ended here, except that one day a close friend asked me to help her with her weight. This led me to organize my thoughts and strategies on paper for the first time. The resulting eight strategies, which I named *The Power of One*, eventually found their way to a weight-loss counselor, who asked if she could adopt them for her clients. Then she said, "You should put these into a book."

My first thought was: "The last thing the world needs is another diet book!" But this quickly changed. The excited reaction of that weight-loss counselor told me I had discovered something important. By figuring out why we are all getting fatter, and how to stop it, I had found a way to bring the nation back to nutritional sanity without imposing any diet on anyone.

From the beginning, though, I realized that if I was going to put what I had discovered into a book, it would have to be unlike any other weight-loss book ever written. I knew that if I just jotted down my strategies, perhaps threw in a few recipes, and padded the pages with facts the average person doesn't want to know, I wouldn't be helping anyone.

You see, I not only wanted to present my eight strategies, I wanted to tell you, the reader, that I know what you are feeling, that I know what you are going through. That I know just how hard it is for you to even *think* about a diet, let alone live one.

Then I wanted to *motivate* you into getting *past* the quick-fix mentality of gimmick diets. To become *excited* about beginning a new life based on *nutritional sanity.* To feel the excitement *I* felt when my own excess weight began to disappear.

And to do all this I needed a new way of conveying my thoughts. That's when I decided to combine my passion for nutrition with my passion for writing fiction.

Using the novel form enabled me to write not just the facts about weight loss, but also to portray the emotional roller coaster all overweight people ride during their weight-loss journey. Through the characters of Fowler, Karen, and Janice, I could explain the strategies I live with, and how I discovered and incorporated them into my life. I was able to show how Karen went from feeling hopeless to hopeful, her inevitable crises, and how she answered the painful question, "Do I have what it takes?"

Even more importantly, I was able to show how The Power of One can be incorporated into your life too, no matter who you are or where you live.

Stephen Moss

WHO IS THIS BOOK FOR?

- *Everyone who is overweight*

  Men. Women. Children over two years old. The slightly overweight and the extremely overweight.

- *Families*

  Who want to get control of their weight and health in a setting that fits all.

- *Understanding nutrition*

  Anyone who wants to understand proper nutrition in a real-life setting.

- *Physicians, dietitians, nutritionists, and fitness professionals*

  Who need an easy to use and understand weight-loss manual for their patients and clients.

- *In short, Lose Weight with The Power of One is for everyone*

Note: *Women who are pregnant, people whose weight gain is directly caused by a psychological or emotional trauma, and those suffering from an eating disorder, should only use this book in conjunction with their health-care provider.*

How To Use This Book

Lose Weight with The Power of One is not a diet book.

Diet books all have certain similarities. First they make your head swim by throwing reams of nutritional jargon at you. Then they give you a set of eating rules to follow. Rules that are inevitably unsustainable. This is when the diet fails.

All diets fail.

Diets fail because they tell you what foods to eat and when to eat them. They fail because they force you to follow someone else's tastes, cravings, and moods.

Diets fail because control of your nutritional lifestyle has been taken from you and put into someone else's hands. Whatever choice you once had over one of life's most basic and enjoyable areas—eating—is gone. And human nature dictates that sooner or later we will refuse to live this way.

Lose Weight with The Power of One takes you in the opposite direction.

This book will empower you. It will not tell you what to eat or when to eat or how to eat. Instead of giving you rules, it presents eight broad guidelines about eating—guidelines that you can pick and choose from depending on your mood, mind-set, or circumstances.

Lose Weight with The Power of One will put the power of control back in your hands, where it belongs. And it will do it in a fun, exciting way. A way designed to quickly motivate you into starting the process.

How to Start

All you need to do is begin reading and let the strength of *Lose Weight with The Power of One* pull you forward. The story of Karen, Fowler, and Janice, along with each of the eight strategies, work together, and should be looked at in their entirety. Only once you have read the whole book through will you have a clear picture of *The Power of One* and the significance of each of the strategies. You can, however, immediately begin incorporating the strategies into your life in any order.

High-fat/Low-fat?

Unlike any diet book, the first strategy of *The Power of One* will tell you how and why to lower your dietary fat, while the last will tell you how and why to raise it. This is because *The Power of One* is neither a high-fat diet nor a low-fat diet. It is not a diet at all. It is knowledge, and with knowledge you can avoid getting caught up in the high-fat/low-fat controversy. *The Power of One* is a sane middle ground: a commonsense program based on the real world.

Definition of Fat-Reduced

Throughout this book you will read the term fat-reduced. The simplest way to illustrate the definition of fat-reduced, is by looking at one of our most common foods: Milk. Milk can be purchased as whole, two percent, one percent, and skim. Each of these variations has less fat content than the one before it. Fat-reduced simply means going down the fat scale one notch at a time, until you reach the level you are comfortable with.

Healthy vs. Unhealthy Foods

Lose Weight with The Power of One will not tell you one food is bad while another is good. It will only point you in the real-life direction of how you can discover the most natural and healthiest way of eating for *your lifestyle*, and not someone else's. You will not need to buy special foods or follow specific recipes.

How to Get the Most Out of This Book

The first time you read *Lose Weight with The Power of One*, the story will grab you. During subsequent readings the eight nutritional strategies will begin to take hold. The book was purposely written this way: in layers, both motivational and practical. Reread the book as often as you need to. The strategies are not there to simply be understood, they are there to become a part of your life. All you need to do is let it happen.

At the end of the book are three appendices. They contain tips and specific information that answer many of the most commonly asked questions about diets and dieting: *Diet Myths, The Energy Bank,* and *Stress*. Following the appendices is a brief overview of each of the eight *Power of One* strategies for easy reference.

If at any point on your journey you hit a "wall," always return to *Lose Weight with The Power of One*. It will serve as the powerful motivational tool you need to get you started again and keep you going until you reach your health and weight-loss goal. Let Karen's journey, with its ups and downs, starts and stops — and ultimate success — encourage you on your own journey.

Now I invite you to sit back, relax, and enjoy *Lose Weight with The Power of One*.

Stephen Moss

The
Power
of One

PROLOGUE

I have been transformed, Karen wrote in her journal. *The Power of One took me from fat to thin. Unhealthy to healthy. Self-conscious to self-confident.*

She paused, reread what she'd just written, then underlined the words *thin, healthy,* and *confident.*

From the back lawn came a shout, then laughter. Karen stepped to the patio door to check on Gabe, her five-year-old, and was about to take her seat again when she caught her reflection in the glass. All she had on was a pair of jeans and a t-shirt, but even after four years she was still thrilled with the way she looked. And it had happened so easily, she thought. Without dieting! Simply by taking one small step, then another, and another.

That was all Fowler had asked of her. An incremental, consistent movement toward better health. Toward losing weight. Let The Power of One slip into your world, he'd said. Let the process be gradual, thoughtful. Let it become a *part* of your life, without intruding *into* your life.

He had talked about courage. Just the amount needed to learn what there was to learn. Then he'd wrapped the eight Power of One strategies within a nest of creativity, promising, "That's all you'll ever need."

And he was right.

Karen smiled, remembering how she'd first resisted, then reluctantly agreed to listen to his words. Only that. Just listen.

And then The Power of One took hold.

"Thank you, Fowler," she whispered. "For showing me the way. For giving me back my life."

She returned to her desk and lifted the pen once again. But instead of writing, she let her mind drift back to how it had all begun.

CHAPTER

1

The screen door slammed behind her. With Gabe crying in her arms, she hurried toward the dark woods at the back of the lawn. After a couple of steps she couldn't catch her breath. By the halfway point she'd slowed to a walk. And at the white oak that marked the beginning of the woods beyond her lawn's boundaries, she stopped, pressed her shoulder against the tree, and fought for air.

The door banged open. Gary stepped onto the porch, belly hanging over the waistband of his red boxers.

Karen, struggling to calm Gabe, turned to face him, thinking, This time he's going to have to beg to get me back! Promise he'll stop calling me names. I know I'm overweight, but that's not the reason for *every* problem.

But Gary yelled, "You can say what you want, Karen! I don't care anymore. You're a fat cow and you make me sick!" And with that he stormed back into the kitchen.

Karen watched through the screen as Gary took a few steps, seemed to change his mind, lifted her purse from where she'd slung it over the back of a chair, then turned to the door again and, purse held high, yelled, "Running into the back wasn't a good idea, Karen, especially without this. 'Cause now I'm locking you out!" Then he slammed the storm door, slid the bolt, and shut the porch light, leaving the yard in blackness.

Karen was stunned. For a moment all she could do was stare at the door. Then she cursed softly, her chest welling with anger and frustration. Taking a deep breath to calm herself, she lowered her head to Gabe's and thought, Okay, Gary, you know I have no place to go. So you're waiting, expecting me to knock at the door, ask to be let in. Even apologize for standing up for myself! But that's not going to happen. I'll stay out all night before I give you that satisfaction!

And with this she turned toward the woods.

In the six weeks she'd lived here she had never before gone beyond the perimeter of the lawn, had not yet found the time to see where her town-house community met the farmhouses and barns of a passing era.

I don't have to go far, she reasoned. Just far enough so Gary will have to search for me when he starts to worry. Force him to bend a little. All I need is a place to sit, and I'll wait him out!

The night was warm, the sky brilliant with stars. Karen, quickly winded again, kept her pace slow and let her rocking motion lull Gabe to sleep. She made her way through the woods until she came to a clearing where a split-rail fence lay forgotten. With Gabe in her lap, she sat next to one of the fence posts. Once more she struggled to regain her breath.

But now a familiar knot fell into place in her gut, one that had been tightening for years, clamping down with each pound gained. She sighed, hating the feeling, and realized that after sixty pounds, the knot had finally twisted into hopelessness.

Then she heard a man's voice call out, "Courage!"

The word, a sudden shout in the night, startled her. It was as if her own spirit were urging her on, demanding strength. It came again: "Courage!" She held her breath, waited for more, then heard, the tone softer now, "Hey, boy. You see something? Is something there?"

A large dog bounded from the trees toward her. It stood barking on the other side of the fence until the voice commanded, "Courage! Get back here!"

The dog instantly obeyed, but the next moment Karen was blinded by a bright beam of light. She lifted her hand to shield her eyes. The light dropped to the ground. Gabe began to cry.

Karen blinked, tried to focus. The light, now held low, moved toward her. She could make out the shadow of a man. He stopped about fifteen feet from where she sat, and once more lifted the light, though this time only until it illuminated the fence and Gabe. With her instincts on edge, Karen waited, thinking, At even a hint of trouble, I'm running!

But the man switched off his flashlight and said a cautious hello. The distance between them was too far for Karen to make out his features. He stepped closer, to just beyond arm's length from the fence, and, dropping to one knee with the dog beside him, said, "Sorry about the light. We didn't know anyone was here. I hope Courage didn't scare you. He wouldn't harm a flea."

"It's okay," Karen answered. "We're fine."

The fence crossed Karen at chest height, creating a buffer. She rocked Gabe, quieting him again, and took a good look at the man.

He was lean. Lithe. Nearing or just past fifty, Karen guessed. His hair was thick and unruly and his cheeks were covered in a day's growth of stubble. He wore a pullover and a dark multi-pocketed vest, and jeans that were tucked into work boots. On his head was a lantern.

The man said, "My name's Fowler, and this is—"

"Courage," Karen said, the word sounding weak coming from her, not at all the way it had sounded when snapped out by the man.

Fowler grinned.

Karen smiled back. Then, realizing that if she could make out Fowler's features so clearly, he could do the same to hers, she immediately lowered her head

It was the thickness of her face she'd grown ashamed of, the roll of her second chin. The swell of fat that had become her waist. She suddenly wished she'd found a cave to hide in and not this clearing, so no one would see she was wearing Gary's old Bulls sweatshirt, because her shirts had again gotten too small, or that she wore sweatpants tagged extra-extra-large, because the only pants or skirts she could get around her were those fitted with elastic waistbands.

"Courage and I were just out gardening," Fowler said.

"Gardening?" Karen again raised her eyes to Fowler's, looking for the joke in his expression, but saw none.

"It's what I do," Fowler said. "Garden. Often at night. Then I write about it in magazines." For a moment the only sound was Courage's breathing. Then Fowler continued, "Lacewing. Lacewing larvae. I was checking how they're doing on the hostas."

"Really," Karen replied, not sure what to make of this conversation.

"Yes. Lacewing larvae. They're a good insect. We buy them — gardeners, I mean — and put them where there're mites. I don't like chemicals. Never have. Don't like anything I can't pronounce."

Karen nodded her head, accepting what he said although she had no idea what it meant.

"I put a whole slew of them on my hostas," Fowler continued, more animated now, "and they've done an excellent job. Better than I expected. And I'm out now because I can see them more clearly at night, the plants and the bugs and what they've done, because of my lights, the intensity of my lights. This one," he said, lifting his flashlight, "and this one too," he added, touching the lamp on his head. Then, lifting it off, holding it slightly toward Karen, he explained, "This is the kind they use in mines. You know, down in the shafts. Keeps your hands free." He smiled broadly. "Works well here too. In my world."

"I would never have thought of that," Karen said. "It sounds like you've got it all worked out."

Courage pushed a wet nose beneath Fowler's chin and nudged his neck. "And Courage likes to come with me," Fowler continued, "to keep me company. Isn't that so, old boy?"

"He's a beauty," Karen said, stretching her arm out so the dog could sniff her hand. "Shepherd, right?"

"Shiloh Shepherd, the biggest, most affectionate Shepherd there is. A really special breed."

Karen gave the black and grey dog a gentle rub behind the ears. "We had a dog when I was growing up. For years she was my best friend." Then she added, "I'm Karen, and this is Gabe. We're your neighbors. From just past the trees. We've been sort of... locked out." She said nothing further and was grateful Fowler didn't ask for details.

Courage whined lightly and again nudged Fowler's neck. Fowler stroked the dog, saying, "You want to go back home, don't you?" Turning to Karen, he added, "His best friend's in the house, and he hates to leave her for very long." He hesitated. "Are you two going to be alright out here?"

"Oh, yes," Karen replied, trying to sound as if she meant it.

Fowler looked unconvinced. "The house is just a stone's throw from here," he said. "The least I can do is offer a locked-out neighbor a chair to sit in and a cup of coffee"

Before Karen had a chance to respond, Fowler stood, propped the flashlight under his chin, and, with a little grunt, lifted the old fence rail off its post and placed it aside, creating a doorway. Then he held out his hand.

CHAPTER

2

Karen reached for Fowler's hand and stood, knowing the first thing he was going to see was her size. The weight that had crept up when she hadn't been looking—weight that now ruled her life the way the black plague had ruled the Dark Ages.

Fowler gestured her forward and she quickly stepped ahead of him, not wanting to catch his expression when he took in the thickness of her waist, the layers of fat on her thighs and buttocks. She held tighter to Gabe, wishing she could be thin the way Fowler was thin. The way she kept promising Gary she'd once again become.

They walked for only a minute, with Courage leading the way and Fowler behind, lighting the path. Karen could see little, but now she began to feel a park-like quality to the land, and to smell, suddenly, the perfume of a thousand flowers. She could sense a freshness here, one missing in the concrete rigidity of her town-house complex.

The path took a sudden turn to the right and widened. The woods came to an abrupt end. Courage ran to a broad sweep of light coming from the back porch of a single-story farmhouse, the building squat, stone solid, with a gable roof and overflowing window boxes. I've stepped back in time, Karen thought, realizing this place was only minutes from her kitchen window, and she'd never known it. She turned to look at Fowler. "This is unbelievable."

"It's out of the way now, sort of hidden, with all the new developments," Fowler said, "but when I first moved in, there were only these old farmhouses."

Karen stepped onto the wide green and white porch and past a stout table flanked by heavy slatted chairs. Fowler, right behind her, reached out and opened the farmhouse's back door.

Courage rushed in first. Karen stepped into a large wood-paneled cloakroom just in time to catch a last glimpse of him as he disappeared through a doorway near the end of a long hall. She turned to Fowler and was surprised to see his expression was now one of resignation. Even determination. He placed his lamps on a wooden shelf and, removing his vest, said, "If you'll excuse me for a moment, I'll just tell my daughter we've got company." He hung his vest on a hook and, stepping from the cloakroom, disappeared around the same corner Courage had taken.

Karen waited with Gabe in her arms, wondering what had caused Fowler's mood to change. She looked around at the neat line of coats and raincoats hanging side by side. At a collection of old terra-cotta pots stacked one into the other. She smiled to herself at a brass coat rack where an assortment of dog leashes shared equal space with a pair of garden clippers.

Gabe stirred in her arms. "I know," she whispered, "you should be in your crib now, not here." Her jaws tightened, the night's argument still fresh in her mind. Can't you even try to understand, Gary, she thought. Do you have to turn every problem into another fight over my weight!

She heard the sound of voices, but they weren't loud enough for her to make out the words. For an instant she thought of just slipping out, then Fowler reappeared. Shaking his head, he said, "Sorry to be so long. Just a little family conference." He motioned toward the door right outside the cloakroom. "Please, go on in. Here's that chair I promised you."

Karen stepped through the doorway, ready to apologize for being here at all, when instead she exclaimed, "What an interesting room."

The space was large, lit by a series of matching wall lamps, their soft light reflecting off the polished oak floor. In the center of the room sat an overstuffed easy chair, along with a television and vcr. In front of the deep bay window, a pine table had begun to curve beneath the weight of dozens of potted plants, many in full bloom, while at the far end of the room stood a magnificent deep green tree in a terra-cotta pot that blocked all but a glimpse of what Karen thought must be the front door.

Motioning toward the tree, Karen said, "Your plants are beautiful."

"One of my passions," Fowler replied. "That's an aralia. I've had it forever. And this," he said, pointing to a green sprout in a tiny clay pot standing on a coffee table next to the easy chair, "is my latest, sent to me from a reader in Arizona. I'm still studying it."

Along with the plant, the coffee table held textbooks and notepads, pencils and chalk, a calculator, a magnifying glass, and an open bag of potting soil.

Karen turned to the wall behind her, where a sofa, seemingly pushed out of the way, was stacked with magazines. But what really held her attention was an old-time schoolhouse blackboard mounted just a foot or so off the floor, entirely banding the wall. Filling the blackboard in small, neat script were line after line of numbers and mathematical symbols.

"Have a seat," Fowler said, pointing to the easy chair. Then, as though noticing it for the first time, he stepped over to the coffee table and placed the bag of potting soil onto the floor.

Karen sank into the large chair, saying, "This is exactly what we needed." She arranged a sleeping Gabe in her lap, then lightly covered his head with a corner of his blanket.

For a moment Fowler stood awkwardly next to her, then with another of his quick grins said, "I'd better clear a space for me too." He stepped to the sofa and rearranged the magazines, then turned to

Karen. "I promised you a coffee, didn't I? There's a fresh pot brewing. I'll be right back."

From behind her, Karen heard the clatter of coffee cups and spoons. Again she heard Fowler speaking and assumed it was with his daughter. She leaned her head back and sighed, wondering if Gary had decided to go look for her yet, or if his stubborn streak still had him parked in front of the tv. She looked about the room again, soaking in its warmth, its endearing oddness. The blackboard told her Fowler was not only an eccentric gardener, but also a scientist of sorts. That he didn't have many visitors was obvious. She wondered too about the daughter, why she hadn't at least stepped in to say hello. Karen sank deeper into the comfortable chair, realizing this was the first time she'd been able to relax in a long while. Why can I do that here, she thought, and not in my own home?

Fowler returned with a tray in his hands. "How do you take it?" he asked, setting the tray onto the table beside her.

"Milk and sugar, please." Karen sat upright, once again adjusting Gabe, and accepted the cup from Fowler. "Thank you so much," she said, "for this and for inviting us in."

"My pleasure," Fowler replied, walking over to the sofa.

Karen took a sip of her coffee. "This is excellent."

Fowler grinned. "My own blend. I buy the beans and grind them myself. I'm not a big coffee drinker, but I like to experiment with it."

Why am I not surprised to hear that, Karen thought, taking another sip. Then she said, "I hope I'm not putting you or your daughter out."

But at that moment Fowler was not looking at her but past her, wearing a pleased, surprised expression. "Speaking of my daughter," he said, "here she is now."

Karen turned to see her, but with the baby and the coffee she couldn't turn quite enough.

Fowler, still looking at his daughter, said, "It's alright... Why don't you join us?"

"I only wanted to see the baby." The voice was not loud, but strong, self-assured, and strangely rough.

Karen set her cup down and looked behind her.

Fowler said, "Karen, this is Janice."

All Karen could see edged past the terra-cotta pot of the large tree was the front of an electric wheelchair. And feet. Tiny feet in white socks poking out from beneath a plaid wool blanket. Feet not much larger than Gabe's.

"Come and say hello," Fowler said. "I'm sure Karen would be happy to show you the baby."

Karen turned back to Fowler. He nodded to her. She faced the girl again, saying, "Of course..." when her words stuck in her throat. The girl had her small hand around the black lever of the chair and had moved herself clear of the tree.

She was no more than three feet tall and sat in the chair at an awkward angle, shoulders slightly hunched. Her features were severely deformed, her skin color bruising shades of red. Karen was shocked. Courage, tail wagging, stood beside the wheelchair.

Karen heard Fowler call her name. She turned to him, eyes still wide.

"Janice has never seen a baby before," Fowler said calmly, his eyes locked on Karen's.

"Except on tv," Karen heard Janice say.

Once more Karen turned to Janice. She forced herself to look directly at her, struggled to regain her composure. Somehow she found the words to say, "You can come closer. It's alright."

Janice inched her chair forward again, stopping it beside the tv. Karen lowered the blanket from Gabe's head and watched as the girl's eyes lit, suddenly thinking, My God, she's got the most beautiful eyes

I've ever seen, so large and green. She moved Gabe so that he faced her, and could not help but smile at Janice's expression of wonder.

Fowler said to Janice, "Can I get you a coffee?"

At this, Janice hesitated.

Karen glanced at Fowler and he gave her the slightest of nods. She turned to Janice. "Yes, please join us."

Fowler stood. "I'll just get you a cup. I'll be right back." He walked over to his daughter, gave her shoulder a quick squeeze, and was out of the room.

In her rough voice Janice asked, "What's the baby's name?"

"Gabe," Karen answered. "He just turned six months." Gabe's eyes were beginning to open. "He's starting to wake up," Karen said. "Why don't you come a little closer, so you can really see him."

Janice touched the lever on her wheelchair, stopping next to the easy chair. Still wearing a look of awe, she whispered, "He's beautiful."

"He is," Karen replied. "I mean, of course I think he is." She laughed lightly.

Fowler returned and handed a cup of coffee to Janice. "How's everything going?" he asked, looking from Janice to Karen.

"Great," Karen said.

Janice smiled at Fowler. Karen could see her eyes glowing.

CHAPTER

3

Fowler again took his seat, this time relaxing fully into it and crossing his legs.

Karen turned to him. He smiled at her but said nothing. Turning back to Janice, she said, "Would you like to touch Gabe?"

"Oh yes," Janice answered.

Karen said to Gabe, "Someone wants to say hello. Her name is Janice." She lifted Gabe, letting his blanket remain in her lap, and placed him in a seated position on the wide arm of the easy chair. "Hi, Janice," she whispered, her face behind Gabe's.

Janice reached out and touched one of Gabe's stockinged feet. Even for her small body, Janice's arms were too short, but Karen could see they were perfectly functional.

Janice said, "Hello, Gabe." Then, looking at Karen, she added, "He's so warm."

"He is. Babies always seem that way. Put one of your fingers into his hand. See what happens."

Janice touched Gabe's palm with her forefinger and Gabe wrapped his fingers around it. Janice laughed.

Karen, though finding the sound unusually rough, couldn't help laughing along with her. Fowler did the same and Karen saw that his expression was now one of absolute pleasure.

"Is he hungry?" Janice asked Karen. Her hand was still firmly in Gabe's grip. Karen could see she was in no hurry to move it from him.

"No," Karen answered. "I think he's going to go back to sleep." For a few moments the three of them watched as Gabe's eyes slowly closed.

Then Fowler said to Karen, "What about you? Are you hungry? Would you like something with your coffee?"

Karen turned to him and thought, That sounds good. Then she gritted her teeth and said to herself, No! I'm not going to eat again until I've lost all my extra weight! Until there's no more reason for Gary to complain.

Janice, glancing at her, asked, "Is anything wrong?"

"No, no. I'm fine," Karen quickly answered.

"My father's a really good cook."

"We'll let Karen decide that for herself," Fowler said, standing. "What'll it be? Something warm? Something cold? Something straight out of the garden? I have it all." He walked to Janice and, standing beside her chair, stared down at Gabe, who was still holding on to Janice's finger.

"Something warm for me," Janice said, momentarily taking her eyes off Gabe to look at her father.

"There's one customer," Fowler grinned, getting a smile from Janice in return.

Karen said, "Nothing for me. Please, don't bother..."

"It's no bother," Janice said. "He'll just take something out of the freezer."

Of course it's no bother, Karen thought. He can eat all he wants and enjoy it. She hesitated for a moment before giving in to her hunger. "Okay, maybe just something small."

"Why don't we go into the kitchen then?" Fowler said to Janice.

Janice nodded her head. With obvious reluctance she pulled her finger from Gabe's grip.

Fowler said to Karen, "We're just going to move to the next room, but I should first tell you—"

"What he should tell you," Janice said, "is to brace yourself."

CHAPTER

4

Karen wrapped Gabe into his blanket and stood. She followed Janice and Courage. Fowler, with their coffees, was just behind her. "This is the last thing I would have expected tonight," Karen said. "All I planned on doing was staying away from home for an hour or so, just until..." But the moment she stepped past the potted tree into the next room, the balance of her sentence was lost. "This is amazing."

Janice said, "It's my father's restaurant."

"This does look like a restaurant, doesn't it?" Karen said.

The first thing she saw was a long polished table and just beyond it a glass-fronted, deli-style counter, softly underlit and curved at its ends to enclose the space behind it. The counter divided the room diagonally into two distinct parts, the eating and cooking areas.

"I always wanted my own restaurant — my kind of restaurant," Fowler said. "But I never needed to make a living from it. So I built it here, in my house." He stepped around the counter into the cooking area.

Karen smiled quizzically and continued to look around the room.

The walls were a combination of bricks and wooden beams, dotted with copper ornaments. Lush green plants hung from copper chains and more trees stood in terra-cotta pots on the floor. The window was framed by red checked curtains.

Lined up neatly inside the serving counter were containers of all sizes, along with milk, a bowl of fruit, and a pot of peeled potatoes in water.

Fowler said, "Come on in and I'll give you the tour."

Karen stepped around the serving counter, as Fowler pointed out the kitchen's features. "Commercial stove, bakery oven, professional mixer, and all the space I could ask for," he said. "Of course, no one needs all this in their house, but I like it."

"He's like a kid in here playing with his toys," Janice said.

"A chef's dream come true," Karen replied in astonishment, looking at the chrome refrigerator and freezer, huge double sink, stainless-steel shelving and counter space, all of it gleaming.

"Why don't you have a seat," Janice said. "The baby must be getting heavy." She pointed to one of four high-backed chairs tucked around the long pine table. Two more chairs, each supporting a green and white palm, stood next to the window.

Karen took a seat. At one end of the table was another collection of books and more papers and pencils.

Janice maneuvered her wheelchair to the head of the table next to Karen, saying, "This is where we spend most of our time." Courage, as though attached to Janice by an invisible leash, stayed at her side.

"If I had this kitchen, I'd never leave it," Karen said. Then, looking at the wall at the nearer end of the kitchen, she said with even more surprise, "What's that?"

On the wall were a pair of men's work trousers, size extra-extra-extra-large, spread wide and mounted in a frame, and on a shelf of its own, as though it was a trophy, a full bottle of Canadian whisky. And, between those two items, an unlit, four-foot, blue neon sign that read, The Power of One.

"The Power of One?" Karen said, turning to Fowler. "What does that mean?"

But Fowler's back was to her, and Janice, her attention again fully on Gabe, said to Karen, "He's fast asleep."

"He is," Karen replied. She continued to examine the room — a tan sofa where none would be expected, and still more plants, each more exotic than the other. Then she turned to Fowler again, this time catching his eyes, and realized that from where he stood he could clearly see her profile. See how Gabe rested on her stomach instead of her lap. How her thighs hung over the sides of the seat. Using the pretext of adjusting Gabe again, she let his blanket fall so that it hid most of her too.

She lowered her head to the top of the baby's and sank into another overwhelming sense of hopelessness, aware of just how much her weight controlled her life. She pictured what she looked like now — big round face, fat body in an old sweatshirt and sweatpants.

"Is there something we can do for Gabe? Janice asked. "Does he need anything?"

At Janice's words Fowler suddenly said, "I'll be right back," and hurried out a door at the far end of the kitchen.

Janice wore an expression that said this type of behavior should be expected from her father. "He's got an answer for every situation."

"I'm beginning to see that."

"I still get surprised," Janice continued, "but this time I can guess where he's going. To get my old cradle from the spare room."

Fowler quickly returned with a wooden cradle and a blanket. "This should do nicely," he said, putting the cradle on the floor behind Karen's chair and giving it a nudge so that it began to rock.

"It's beautiful," Karen said, admiring the rich, dark wood.

"We bought it just before Janice was born," Fowler said, holding out his hands for Gabe. Karen handed him the sleeping baby, and Fowler gently placed him into the cradle. He watched Gabe for a moment, then again stepped behind the counter.

Karen, leaning to Janice, asked, "May I use your bathroom?"

"Of course," Janice said. "It's just outside there." She pointed to the door Fowler had used.

When Karen returned she saw that Janice had turned her wheelchair so she could watch Gabe. "He moves a lot when he sleeps," Janice said. Courage was stretched out on the floor beside Janice's chair. He thumped his tail as Karen took her seat.

On the table were three fresh coffees and three glasses of water with lemon wedges. Fowler was taking an assortment of cellophane-wrapped items from the freezer. He removed the wrappings and placed their contents in a plastic container, then put the container into the microwave oven and set the timer. Stepping back to the table with a bowl of fruit, he said to Karen, "I'm a night owl, so this is no bother for me."

"He likes to work at night and sleep in," Janice said. "The opposite of me."

"It's true," Fowler explained. "I do my best work long after the sun's gone down." He grinned at Janice. "At least our hours cross during part of the day, so we get the chance to argue about politics." He left the table again, returning with napkins, plates, and forks, then stood next to Janice's wheelchair, as though wondering what else he could do.

The microwave beeped. Fowler went behind the counter and opened the oven's door. Almost immediately Karen could smell the delicious aroma of the snacks he'd prepared, and the first thing she thought was, Here I go again. Ready to stuff my face. And then, Oh God, what am I doing? What am I doing to my marriage! Searching for anything to take her mind off these thoughts, she said to Fowler, "All those diplomas on the wall... Just outside the kitchen... You must be some sort of doctor?"

"No," Fowler said, placing the food on a platter, "those are Janice's. She has a Ph.D. in genetics."

"What?" Karen turned to Janice, instantly regretting her tone and look of surprise.

"There are ways it can be done without leaving the house," Janice said. "There's also a wall in our den filled with my father's plaques, for horticulture and writing. I may have earned my Ph.D., but it was only after he taught me *how* to earn it. How to think things through. How to believe I could do anything I put my mind to, if I only found the courage."

Karen, realizing that every assumption she'd had about Janice had just been shattered, was at a loss for words. But it was more than that, she knew. It was also what Janice had said, about being able to do anything, if only she found the courage. *Courage.* This was the second time tonight that word had struck her.

Fowler stepped up to the table with the snacks. On the platter were meatballs, bite-size pizza wedges, and strips of chicken covered in cheese. He placed the platter on the table and took his seat.

Karen, leaning back in hers, again glanced at Janice, then once more lifted her eyes to the sign that read, The Power of One.

CHAPTER

5

Before reaching for any of the snacks, Karen sighed, knowing what she had to do. She turned to Janice and said, "I'd better call home. Can I use your phone?"

"Of course." Janice again pointed toward the door that led to the hallway. "It's just outside, on a small table."

Karen left the room. She tried to summon anger and failed. She found trepidation instead. Gary picked up the phone on the first ring and said, "Where the hell are you?"

She tried to explain, tried to keep her voice calm, but Gary replied angrily, "You're pushing me too far, Karen."

"Gary, please," Karen said, just before he slammed down the phone.

Damn you, Karen thought, why do you have to be so stubborn! All I did was stick up for my rights. She returned to the kitchen and took her seat. For a few seconds there was an embarrassed silence. Then Janice, with an expression of concern, asked, "Is everything okay?"

Karen pressed her lips to a line. "My husband Gary's hot-tempered, and once he gets fired up, it takes him a while to cool down."

"That can't be easy."

"It isn't." Karen reached for a wedge of pizza and held it, adding, "We've been arguing for months now, ever since the baby was born. I wish there was something I could do—just snap my fingers and make everything better. But I can't. And I can't even put all the blame on Gary, because it's my fault too."

"What do you mean?" Janice asked.

Karen took a bite of the pizza and pointed at the platter of snacks. "This is the problem. My weight. No matter how the argument begins, it always ends up being about that—the fact that I have no self-control."

To Karen's surprise Fowler said, "That's not true."

"No. That isn't the way it works," Janice added.

But Karen, feeling a fresh rush of emotion, put the balance of the pizza wedge onto her plate and said, "It's ruining our marriage, making him hate me. But I try!"

"I'm sure you do," Janice said sympathetically.

Karen turned to Fowler for an instant and then back to Janice. "And then sometimes I think he's supposed to love me for who I am. The person inside this fat body. Why do *I* have to struggle to lose weight? Live on lettuce and carrots for the rest of my life? He wouldn't do it. I know him."

"Have you tried telling him that?" Janice asked, placing her small hands on the table. "The way you just told me."

"I'm not telling him anything," Karen said. "He locked me out, can you believe it? Locked me and his son out of the house, just because I can't get my weight under control." She looked into Janice's eyes, then sighed. "I'm sorry. I'm sure you don't want to hear this."

"I'm a good listener," Janice said.

Karen reached out and touched her hand. Then, taking a deep breath, she said, "But it's time for me to leave."

"Where will you go?"

Karen had no answer.

Fowler said, "I can give you a lift somewhere, if that'll help."

"Maybe that will help," Karen said. Standing again, she added, "We've only been here a short time, just since Gary's transfer, and we don't know many people yet. But I have a friend at work—Sue. We've

gotten quite close. I'm sure she'll let me spend the night at her place."
She gestured that she'd be back in a moment and again went to the
telephone. But after seven long rings she put the phone down and
walked back into the kitchen. She shook her head, saying, "There's no
answer," and remained standing, not looking forward to a night in the
woods, no matter how safe it was.

But Janice quickly cut into those thoughts. "Then why don't you
stay here?"

"Would that be alright?" Karen asked.

"Of course it's alright," Fowler said, sliding back his chair and
standing. "The spare room's all set up. I'll just go get some blankets,
then come back for Gabe." He stepped from the room.

"Thank you," Karen said to Janice. "I wasn't planning on being
anyone's houseguest."

Janice smiled. "It's our pleasure." She nudged the lever on her
chair, saying, "Come, I'll show you where the room is."

CHAPTER

6

Karen awoke to the morning sun shining through sheer curtains. It took a moment for her to orient herself, to realize that this small neat room with its double bed and maple bureau was in Fowler's house. She looked over the side of the bed to see Gabe in the cradle, staring back at her, and whispered, "Good morning." Then she sighed and replayed the events of the night before.

She was thankful it was Monday, so she didn't have to work and Gary did. When she got home, he would already be gone. For an instant she wondered if she would still be locked out, then dismissed that thought. Gary might be insensitive about her weight, but he wasn't vengeful. Still, she was not looking forward to seeing him.

Then her thoughts shifted to who she was with, her unusual neighbors, and to a renewed appreciation for Janice.

At Gabe's cry, she swung her legs off the side of the bed, remembering how graceful she'd been when she was sixty pounds lighter. She lifted Gabe into her arms and pressed her lips against his cheek, whispering, "I love you." Then she carried him over to the window and drew aside the curtain.

Fowler's garden was an immaculate sweep of color. Deep blues, intense reds. A painting of flowerbeds and winding pathways screened by a dense curtain of shrubbery and trees. Her eyes widened at both the vista and its seclusion. What she was seeing was only minutes from her own backyard, but completely hidden from view. It's true, she thought, he has created a world of his own.

She turned from the window and caught her reflection in a mirror fastened onto the bedroom door. Once again she felt the knot in her gut tighten.

All she could see was a pear-shaped figure with a heavy double chin. You're right, Gary, she thought. It's me. I'm fat. You married someone thin, and no matter how I try, I can't change back. But she forced these thoughts from her mind, knowing she had to get home as soon as possible to change and feed Gabe.

She opened the door to the room. On a chair in the hall was a stack of diapers. I don't believe this, she thought.

"Good morning," Janice said when Karen, with a freshly changed Gabe in her arms, stepped into Fowler's restaurant.

This morning Janice wore a crisp white blouse. Instead of her blanket she had on a long blue skirt that ended at her tiny feet. She touched the lever on her wheelchair and tucked herself at the table. A newspaper was spread out and another book filled with mathematical symbols was open amid papers covered with her neat script. At the back of the room, Courage busily ate from a bowl set on a shelf a foot off the floor.

"Good morning," Karen said. Then, seeing what else was waiting for her, she added, "Oh no. He shouldn't have..."

At the other end of the table were assorted jars of baby food and cereal, a bottle, colored spoons, and a baby seat.

"I'll pay him back as soon—" Karen began.

"Don't bother trying," Janice said. "He won't take your money."

"How could he even have thought of this?" Karen asked. "Gary would never have figured it out." She reached for a jar of food and the spoons.

"Fowler's not typical," Janice said, watching as Karen began to feed Gabe. "He's always been ahead of the curve."

"What does that mean?" Karen asked, noticing that Janice's voice didn't sound quite as harsh to her ear as it had the night before.

"It means he has this ability to be a half-dozen steps ahead of everyone else, in whatever field interests him. Whether it's gardening or nutrition or philosophy." Janice reached out and touched the baby's foot, holding it for a moment with another expression of delight.

Karen smiled, then glanced at the book on the table and read out the title, *Triangulating an n-Dimensional Cube.*

"One of my hobbies," Janice said. "Trying to work out unsolved mathematical problems. I like the way they twist my mind, take me away from genetics. My father calls the work I do on the blackboard in the living room 'Chinese cooking.'"

Karen laughed. "It looks that way to me too." Then, her eyes falling once again on the sign on the wall, she asked, "What's The Power of One?"

For a moment Janice didn't reply, then she said, "It's a way of life. Something my father developed."

"A way of life?" Karen repeated, wiping a spill from Gabe's chin.

Janice nodded. "Actually, it's more something that *fits into your life, without disrupting it.*" Then she said, "You know, you're the first person to ever ask what it means."

"What?" Karen said. "How could anyone see that sign and not ask what it means?"

Janice closed the newspaper and put it aside. "Because no one else has ever seen it. We don't have many visitors. In fact, we don't have any." Then she quickly said, "The Power of One—I must have begun hearing that phrase when I was eleven or twelve, maybe fifteen years ago."

"You're... twenty-seven?"

"Twenty-six."

Karen stared at Janice for a moment. Then looked at the sign again, and at the trousers. "Were those your father's?"

Janice nodded.

"You mean, he was once that fat?"

Again Janice nodded.

Karen shook her head. "I don't know how some people do it. Go on a diet and lose all their weight, and keep it off. I start a new diet every few months..."

"—Diets aren't the answer," Janice said. "That's not how he lost his weight. Look in the cupboard behind you."

Karen offered Gabe a final spoonful of food, which he refused. Then she turned and opened the cupboard behind her chair. Inside were six shelves tightly packed with books. With just a glance at the titles she could see they were all diet books.

"Fowler's read every one of them," Janice said, "sometimes because he wanted to lose weight, and sometimes because he just wanted to see what new gimmick was currently making the rounds."

"I also read a lot of these books," Karen said. "And I'm still over-weight."

"That's because diets don't work," Janice answered. "And the reason they don't work is because their approach is wrong. They try to tell you what to do, put you into the diet mentality of anxiety and guilt."

"Then what does work?"

"Just basic information," Janice said, "beginning with *why* you're overweight, and *how to protect yourself from that*. But I'd better let Fowler tell you about it. He has a knack for taking complexities and turning them into simple, commonsense truths—in a way most people can't."

CHAPTER

7

"**G**ood morning," Fowler said, stepping into the restaurant and tipping his head.

"Thank you for all this," Karen said, indicating the baby supplies on the table.

"My pleasure," Fowler replied, walking to the cooking area. "Tea or coffee?"

"Coffee." Janice answered.

"Coffee for me too," Karen said, adding, "But I should be going soon. I know Gary will be waiting to hear from me."

"You can always call him from here," Janice said.

"No. I don't think so. I don't know what to expect, and if he's still upset, I'd rather hear it at home. This isn't the place to get another insult about my weight." She sighed. "He calls my weight his punishment for having met me."

Janice said, "He can't mean that."

"He does. And maybe he's right." What Karen didn't say was that last night Gary had also called her lazy and stupid, and that that was the reason she'd walked out. Karen shook her head. "I'm just not able to get my weight under control, no matter how hard I try. Even *I* think there must be something wrong with me."

"There's nothing wrong with you," Janice protested.

Karen ignored her words and continued. "I know I'm a bright woman, and for three days a week I handle a responsible job. I tell that to myself. Then I hear Gary, or just step in front of a mirror, and I know there must be something wrong."

Fowler brought three coffees to the table and went back behind the counter.

"I *will* lose the weight, though, I know it," Karen said. But even as Janice began to nod in agreement, she added, "No. I won't. I've tried enough times to know it'll never come off. For me, losing weight is only a dream. I'm someone who doesn't even have to eat to gain extra pounds. Just the smell of burgers and fries does it. And I can't go on another diet. I can't even face that thought."

Fowler returned to the table with three glasses of water with lemon wedges.

Karen said, looking at him, "Janice said you were once fat too."

Fowler sat and leaned back in his chair. "No. I'm still fat. What you're looking at is a fat person in a thin body. And I'm proud to be that way. Not ashamed to say I have a weight problem."

Janice smiled, but Karen looked bewildered.

Fowler said, "I weigh myself every morning."

"So do I," Karen replied.

I know you do," Fowler said. "And like you, I also gain weight with just the smell of burgers and fries. But I have the problem under control."

"Because of that?" Karen asked, pointing to the sign. "The Power of One?"

Fowler nodded.

"The Power of One isn't a diet," Janice said, "but it did solve his weight problem."

"I used The Power of One to think it all through," Fowler said, "carefully and commonsense-fully. I defined the problem, and learned the information I needed to solve it."

Karen said, "I'd love to not have to diet again. When I was thirty pounds overweight, I starved myself down fifteen pounds — then gained back twenty! Then I lost the twenty on a protein diet because that's all everyone was talking about—"

"Well, you know *that* won't work," Janice said.

"You're right," Karen agreed. "When I couldn't stand not being able to eat half the foods I loved, I gained the twenty back — and more!" She took one last sip of her coffee, and stood, saying, "I'm sorry, but I really have to go."

"Will you come back?" Janice said.

"Yes. I'd like that."

"You can bring Gabe," Janice said. "We can talk again."

Fowler, also standing, said, "How about tomorrow? Can you come over for lunch?"

After only a second's hesitation, Karen said, "Lunch sounds perfect."

CHAPTER

8

This time Karen took the side street that joined her development to the old two-lane highway running past Fowler's front door. The day was warm and the sky clear, but her thoughts about Gary were anything but sunny.

He'd telephoned from work only minutes after she got into the town-house. At first he was repentant, apologizing for losing his temper, promising it would never happen again. But after asking about the neighbors she'd stayed with, and hearing about Fowler's eccentricities and Janice's condition, and then about the sign on the wall, he'd blown up again, saying, "You don't know what kind of life that makes them live. How could you have stayed there?"

He'd been unrelenting, not letting Karen get in a word, and had ended the conversation by shouting, "If you want to walk the streets, do it! If you want to go to some flea bag hotel, you can do that too! But you keep my son away from people like that!"

Last night at home, he'd been silent.

It was only as she came up Fowler's front walk, though, that Karen realized what was bothering her most. It wasn't Gary's words, but his tone. A tone, she felt, that should not be part of any marriage.

Fowler opened the door and welcomed her. She lifted Gabe from his stroller and Fowler held out his hands for him. Janice, smiling broadly, also gave her a warm hello.

They went to the kitchen, and Karen was surprised how wonderfully at home she suddenly felt. But as Fowler strapped Gabe into his seat on the table, she took her cell phone from her bag and said, "If I get a call, please don't listen to what I'm going to say, because I'm not supposed to be here."

"If your husband calls, say whatever you have to and don't worry about us," Janice said.

Fowler agreed, then asked, "What would you like for lunch? Any requests?"

"Why don't I just leave it up to you," Karen said.

"Sounds good to me," Fowler replied, stepping into the cooking area.

Karen walked up to the counter. "Can I help you with anything?"

"Oh, an assistant. Now that's an offer I never refuse."

At the table, Janice touched Gabe on the arm and said to him, "Hello, beautiful little man," and was treated to a wide, toothless smile. Once again she had an assortment of math books and papers on the table, but for the moment she ignored them.

Fowler grinned at Karen and said, "Looks like Gabe's found a new friend." Then he filled two glasses with water and put a wedge of lemon into both. Handing one to Karen, he said, "How about something quick and easy, one of my favorites. A stir-fry with fried potatoes, sort of."

"Sort of?"

"You'll see what I mean."

"Sounds good to me," Karen said. "Anything fried, especially potatoes, and I'm in there. Just tell me what to do."

"Okay. Why don't you start with the spuds. Say about twelve."

From the table Janice said, "Twelve potatoes for three people? I guess we're in for some of my father's kind of cooking."

Karen smiled quizzically.

Fowler told her to peel the potatoes, then cut them into irregular shapes about an inch around.

She nodded and got down to work, but, glancing at the sign on the wall again, couldn't resist saying, "You talked about The Power of One—and said it wasn't a diet. But I still don't know what it *is*."

Fowler had put up a large pot of water to boil, switched on the oven, then taken out two packages of chicken breasts from the fridge. Now he was trimming off all the skin and visible fat from the chicken. "The best way to describe The Power of One," he said, "is to compare it to a tire, like one of the tires on my old car. But instead of an engine making this tire roll, its power comes from a tiny pulse of courage."

Courage again, Karen thought.

"And that tiny pulse of courage," Fowler continued, "gets the tire rolling, moving us forward along the road we want to follow. Then another tiny pulse of courage zaps it again, taking us even further, moving us ahead in s*mall forward steps*, until we reach our ultimate goal."

"And we all have The Power of One in us," Janice added.

"We do," Fowler replied. "But that doesn't mean we can all reach in and bring it out." Seeing that Karen had finished peeling and cutting the potatoes, he said, "Now drop them into the boiling water for a few minutes, just until you can easily pierce them with a fork. Then put the pot into the sink and run cold water into it to stop the cooking process."

While she was doing this, Fowler diced the chicken breasts, then spiced them with salt, pepper, garlic and Dijon mustard.

"If we all have The Power of One in us," Karen asked, "then why is it that only some of us will be able to get it out?"

"Because," Fowler answered, "The Power of One is based on *knowledge*. And there are some people who'll find that knowledge on their own, while others will simply learn it from those who already have it.

"But most people are so busy just getting from one day to the next that they don't have the time or energy to do either. And without the right knowledge, they can't possibly go forward and complete whatever journey they've begun."

Karen's brow was furrowed. She tested her potatoes, saw they were done, carried the pot to the sink, then opened the cold water and let it run into the pot. While Fowler took both green and red peppers from the fridge, she said, "I'm not sure what you mean by journeys."

"When I talk about journeys, I mean our journeys in life," Fowler said, washing and dicing the peppers. "And for me, taking a journey, like stopping smoking or drinking or—"

"Eating?" Karen said.

"No. We all have to eat. What you mean is losing weight. And that's the first journey I took. And that's what I think of most when I talk about The Power of One."

"He calls that journey a war," Janice said, her finger now in Gabe's hand.

"That's right," Fowler said. "A war — one that can be won only through knowledge." He snapped his fingers and quickly took two large, nonstick frying pans from the cupboard. He sprayed them liberally with nonstick cooking spray and put them onto a medium heat.

"A war won through knowledge," Karen repeated.

"That's right," Fowler said, placing the chicken into one of the pans. Then, turning to her, he added, "Now you can drain your potatoes and drop them into this other pan, and we'll get it all going."

Once the potatoes were in the pan, Fowler spiced them with salt, pepper, garlic, and paprika and tossed them until they were evenly coated and lightly fried. Then, with a flourish, he poured them from the frying pan onto a large, nonstick baking sheet and put the sheet into the oven. After this he added the diced peppers to the chicken and said, "These will cook with the chicken, while the potatoes get the crunch I like. And then we'll eat."

Seeing Karen's puzzled expression, he said, "The trouble most people have with fighting the war to lose weight, to regain their health, is that *they don't know they're in a war*. And if they do realize there's a war going on around them, then *they don't know who the enemy is*. And if they get a feel for the enemy, then they don't have the *information they need to defeat him*."

Karen said slowly, "The Power of One is the pulse of courage, which, combined with the right information, lets you defeat your enemy."

"Exactly."

Karen's expression grew suddenly somber. "Well, in my case, with my war against being fat, I know who the enemy is. Me."

"You're not your own enemy," Janice said.

"Janice is right," Fowler said. "When it comes to being overweight, *no one is their own enemy*." But he ended this line of conversation by saying, "Let's eat," and asked Karen to set the table, telling her where the cutlery and napkins were kept. "We'll also need refills of our water with lemon wedges," he added.

While Karen set the table, Fowler took down three plates and served a reasonable portion of the chicken into each, leaving most of the chicken he'd cooked still in the frying pan. Then he did the same with the potatoes, leaving most of them on the baking sheet.

From the refrigerator he took out a bag of store-bought prewashed greens, poured a good serving into three salad bowls, added a fat-reduced dressing, and said to Karen, "Looks like we're ready." Together they brought the plates to the table.

Karen lifted Gabe in his baby seat, kissed the top of his head, and placed him on one side of the large table, while Janice gathered her books and papers into a neat pile and set them aside.

Fowler sat and said to Karen, "Eat. Dig in. You're not going to find any formality in my restaurant."

Karen, filling her fork with the stir-fry, said, "I want to thank you for inviting me." Then she tasted the stir-fry and added, "This is delicious."

"It's one of our standards," Janice said. "Something we always enjoy."

"A mix-and-match deal," Fowler explained. "One of those things you throw together without much thought, with whatever's on hand. Peppers, onions, mushrooms. Chicken, turkey, veal. Leftover or not. Cooked or raw. I like it because it's quick and always tasty, and I can make a lot of it at a time."

Karen nodded, but her mind was on the potatoes Fowler had prepared. She said, holding one up with her fork, "These are really good."

"Thank you," Fowler answered. "They're one of my favorites. My unfried french fries."

"They do taste like fries, don't they?" Karen said. "Only better. Tangier."

"He makes them by the bagful," Janice said, "then freezes them on a tray so he can put them frozen into a container and take out just the amount he wants, whenever he wants. We both love them. For breakfast, lunch, and dinner."

"Snacks too," Fowler added. "I can eat them cold—or warm them in the microwave. Potatoes are a gift of the gods, and meant to be eaten as often—"

But before he could finish his sentence, Gabe, staring at Janice, let out a sudden, smile-filled squeal.

Janice laughed with obvious delight.

Fowler laughed along with her.

Courage stood and barked.

The cell phone rang.

CHAPTER
9

It was three days before Karen again saw Fowler and Janice. Once more she stood on their back porch with Gabe in her arms. The porch light was off, the back of the house dark.

She hated being here like this, but hadn't known what else to do.

Gary's attitude had grown worse. She'd tried to understand him, told herself his anger was temporary, because of the pressures of his new job, the new house, the baby.

But he refused to discuss it. Told her he was tired of talking.

When he'd called her cell phone during lunch, the first words he'd said were, "Where are you—and don't lie to me!"

"Gary."

"You're back there, aren't you?"

"I'm sorry," she said quickly, but the connection went dead.

She left then, knowing that for her marriage's sake she would not be seeing Fowler and Janice again.

What followed next was something that had never happened before. Three days of silence interrupted by insults.

She did what she had to — her job, the housekeeping, looking after Gabe. She waited for Gary to come around. Saw he was being unreasonable. Tried to talk to him, without success.

Then tonight, while Gary was in the recliner watching baseball on tv and she sat on the sofa reading, he'd said to her, "What's wrong with you? Can't you figure out what the problem is?" He muted the volume on the television.

"I know what the problem is," Karen said, turning to look at his own thick, round face.

"Oh? You do? And what is it?"

"The problem is me."

"Well, you're right there."

"The problem is I can't take care of myself. Of my weight. I know that." Then she said, "And I can't find any courage."

"Courage? What do you mean? Courage to do what?"

"I don't know. Something. Everything." It was *this* word that had stuck with her. Out of all that Janice and Fowler had said, this was the word that continually ran through her mind. *Courage.* A tiny amount of courage, *just enough to take you to the next step.*

She could see Gary's anger build, his thick chest and arms tense. She shook her head and thought, I may not be the same woman you married, Gary, but you're not the same man either. That man began to pack his things after Gabe was conceived. And left by the time he was born.

She took a deep breath. "If there's something wrong with me, Gary, then what about you? You chose me. And had a baby with me."

Courage put his nose against the screen. Karen whispered, "Courage." Then Fowler stepped up, clearly surprised to see her.

"I'm sorry," she whispered.

"Don't be," he said. "It's alright."

He led her into the house and placed Gabe into the baby seat. Karen heard Janice call from down the hall and Fowler went to her.

He returned in just a few minutes, followed by Janice in her wheelchair. She was wearing pajamas. Her expression was a mixture of happiness and unease.

Fowler put the kettle on for tea.

Stopping her wheelchair next to Karen, Janice said, "Do you want to talk about it?"

Karen shook her head. She was fighting back frustration and anger and wasn't sure which emotion fit where. She said to Janice, "I just want to thank you for being here."

"That's what friends are for," Janice answered.

She woke before either Janice or Fowler. Again waiting on the kitchen table were an assortment of baby supplies. She stared at them a moment, then began to look for a paper and pencil.

Janice steered her chair into the room.

Karen turned to her. "I was going to just sneak out," she said. "Leave a thank-you note." She'd gained weight in the past three days, felt bloated and tired.

"Sneak out? Why?" Gabe stretched his hands toward Janice, and she said excitedly, "He recognizes me!"

Karen nodded. She was dreading her next words.

Janice, clearly sensing something was wrong, again asked, "Why were you going to sneak out? Is it because you're afraid of Gary?"

"No, of course not."

"Then what is it?"

Karen sighed. "I'm not afraid of Gary. I'm afraid of losing him. And he's upset with me because I was here. Because I came back here... And now I'm back again."

Janice, looking directly at Karen, said, "Please, have a seat for a minute. There's something I want to say."

Karen, with Gabe in her arms, sat at the table.

"You've said your marriage is in trouble because of your weight," Janice said.

"It is. Gary hates it."

"Alright then. My father's found a way to solve that problem."

Karen winced, then shook her head, feeling herself thud into a new bout of hopelessness at just the thought of another diet. Another failure. After a moment's silence, she said, "I can't. I'm not ready. Not prepared." She knew she had to psych herself up first. Be in a state of mind to push her willpower to the limit. To not eat carbohydrates or fat or any of the foods she craved for as long as possible—until she slipped—then fell.

"But you need it now," Janice said.

Fowler, in his bathrobe, walked into the room.

Janice turned to him and said, "Karen says she's not ready for The Power of One. That she's not sure about it."

For a moment Fowler remained quiet. Then he said to Karen, "I would rather hear you say you're not sure about it than hear you say you're gung-ho and can't wait to have your life changed. That shows me you've got a healthy amount of skepticism."

Janice looked as though she wanted to say something, but didn't.

"On the other hand," Fowler continued, "the only thing we've told you was that to win the war against being fat, all you're missing is knowledge. Knowledge we have. And that's all there is. No magic pill. Nothing to buy." He shrugged. "So maybe your hesitation has less to do with good, healthy skepticism, and more to do with something else."

Karen's jaws tightened. She took a deep breath, felt her anger well, and thought, Why are you pressuring me, Fowler! If I want to go on a diet, I'll do it myself. My way!

Then she thought, They just don't understand.

Karen sighed. "Fowler, unlike you, I'm the type of person who fails at diets. Always. That's why I'm so fat. So if you try to teach me what you know, I won't understand what you're saying, or I won't be able to do whatever it is you expect of me. I won't be able to stick with it. And I'll fail again. And this time I'll not only disappoint myself and Gary, but also you."

Janice, still sitting with her brow creased in thought, said, "Are you saying, then, that you're afraid to simply listen and learn about The Power of One, because you're afraid you'll fail at it?"

"Janice, we have to respect Karen's decision," Fowler said.

"You might have to," Janice answered, "but I don't." Her husky voice suddenly rose as she said to Karen, "Do you know I was supposed to be dead twenty-six years ago? And then, after twenty-five or thirty operations before I turned five, my father was still told my chances of seeing ten were nonexistent. And that even now the best the doctors can do is say they don't know why I'm still here, that my father should be prepared for me to not wake up tomorrow morning or the one after that.

"And can you imagine how it feels to look the way I do, to have to hide in this house? To know I'll never have a husband, a child, the way you do? Never have even a chance at that kind of life, that kind of love?"

Janice shook her head. "My father says I should respect your decision to not try to take control of your situation, to not show the strength your son, your perfect baby boy, should be able to rely on. Well, I don't respect it. In fact, it makes me livid to think that *just the thought of failure* is enough to stop anyone from having the courage to take a step forward."

She dropped her eyes, then lifted them defiantly and shouted, "You said you wanted to sneak out. Well, go!" And with that she backed her chair from the table and maneuvered herself from the room.

CHAPTER

10

Karen sat motionless after Janice had left. Fowler too looked stunned. He said, "She never told me that before."

Karen was breathing heavily, as though she'd been running. She lowered her head, felt shame, and suddenly realized what hopelessness *really* meant. She lifted her eyes to Fowler. He was still staring at the door. She whispered to him, "Please watch Gabe," and, handing the baby to him, went to find Janice.

Janice was in the den she shared with Fowler, facing the curtained window flanked by their two large desks, each a jumble of papers and books, a computer and accessories and snakes of cables.

To her right was a wall filled with Fowler's gardening plaques and ribbons. The other walls held bookshelves crammed with texts and magazines and bound manuscripts.

"Janice," Karen whispered.

Janice said nothing. Made no movement.

"Janice, I'm sorry."

Janice slowly turned her chair around.

"I never meant to hurt you," Karen said. "I was only being honest, and weak, and I'm sorry."

In a still angry but even voice, Janice said, "Sorry? For whom? For me? Or yourself? Because if it's for me, don't be. I long ago accepted that I can't change my appearance, so I ignore it, and work on what I can change — my health, my mind. Because, as human beings, that's what we do. That's our function. Beyond the genetic level of reproducing, *our function in this life is to progress* — physically, intellectually, and spiritually. No matter what, we can't stand still."

"I know you're right," Karen said, her eyes filling with tears.

"I used to look at The Power of One as complete in itself," Janice continued. "But I was wrong. I see that now. There's a step outside The Power of One that has to be taken first. A step we have to provide for ourselves, from within."

Karen wiped her eyes. "It's... fear," she said. "Repeated failure. That's what's holding me back." The one word that kept swirling through her mind was *courage*. She lowered her head, took a deep breath, then in a small voice, whispered, "Help me, Janice."

They returned together. Gabe was in his baby seat, Fowler seated in front of him. To her father Janice said, "Karen asked me to help her take the first step to The Power of One."

Fowler nodded, but Karen could see his concern was still for Janice. He questioned her with his eyes until he was satisfied with what he saw, and only then did he allow himself to relax and say, "Asking for your help *is* the first step."

Karen looked at him. "You mean I've taken the first step?"

"Of course. Asking for help is the *necessary* first step to The Power of One. The first step to finding the information." Again he looked at Janice, then he stood and walked behind the counter and put the kettle on the stove.

Karen lifted Gabe into her arms, as Janice steered her wheelchair to the table.

Fowler prepared three teas and three glasses of water with lemon wedges and brought them to the table on a tray. He too took his seat. For a moment the only one who spoke was Gabe. This time, though, his babbling was ignored.

Then Karen, looking at Fowler, said, "I'll try to make The Power of One work. Try as hard as I've ever tried anything."

She was being honest, she knew. But not forthright. And that was the best she could do. She'd try. She had no faith she would succeed.

She held up a spiral-bound notebook Janice had just given her. "Janice said I should start a journal—about The Power of One. I'm going to write it all down. I'm going to try to understand what it is."

Fowler said, "The Power of One is as simple as your *abc's*. Once you begin, it'll pull you along. Just let it happen. Take in the information, go where the information points, listen to your head, and you can't fail."

Karen began to say, "I've dieted—"

"Let me say it again," Fowler said. "*The Power of One is not a diet — and it does not require a diet mentality*. It's just a bunch of words that will show you how to *look* at your weight in a different way, from a different angle. It will show you *why* you've lost control over your weight and don't even know it. Why all you know is that you're getting fat. That the whole country's getting fat.

"After I've explained it to you, you'll see for yourself that you can't do The Power of One wrong, because with The Power of One everything is *right*. And you can't go off The Power of One, because it's not something you're *on*. And you will never have to start The Power of One over, because it *can't end*. Once you start it, it can't end. Ever."

"It really isn't a diet, is it?" Karen said.

"No, The Power of One isn't a diet. Its goal isn't even to lose weight, though you *will lose all the weight you need to*. What The Power of One really does is return control of your health to where it belongs—in your hands."

Karen, nodding her head, thought, You make it sound so easy. Just listen to your words—and lose weight. But that's impossible—isn't it? She laughed lightly, then said, "Okay, how do we start?"

"We start," Fowler said, "the way we start every morning. With breakfast."

CHAPTER

11

Karen, placing Gabe into his seat, said to Fowler, "This time I'm not *asking* if I can help prepare breakfast."

"And this time," Janice said, "I'll officially baby-sit." She reached for a plastic turnip Fowler had bought for Gabe and held the toy out to the baby.

Karen stepped behind the counter with Fowler, thinking, I'll do my best to learn The Power of One—and fail later. And knowing that in advance will take all the pressure and struggle out of it. She also thought of the call she'd inevitably get from Gary when she got home, but for the moment pushed that from her mind.

"In the restaurant world," Fowler began, "there's a certain protocol that has to be followed. And it goes like this: I'm the chef, so I'm the boss. And starting now, you're the *sous-chef,* and that's French for 'when you work here, you're the gofer.'"

Karen laughed. "That's fine with me."

"Good. Now there's something else I have to tell you, and it's about The Power of One."

"Okay."

"You see, I may know my stuff—I should, I've been learning and living it for the better part of two decades—but that doesn't mean I know how to teach it, so what I'm going to do is a lot of lip-flapping. About everything. And we'll see where that gets us."

Karen smiled and nodded.

"Now to our first order of business," Fowler said, looking over at Janice. "My staff and I need to know what you want for breakfast."

"Something fast and simple," Janice said, "because Karen has to go home and talk to her husband — and then arrange to come back later for lunch."

"You can count on that," Karen answered.

"So, what do you want?" Fowler asked again.

"French toast."

"I love French toast," Karen said. "So does Gary. That's both of our problems. Bread."

Fowler said, "I'll talk to you about bread, but not right now. All you need to know now is that there's *no such thing as a problem food.*" Then, before Karen could question this, he rapidly said, "Okay, okay. We need eggs, milk, and bread. Let's go, let's go, there's a hundred hungry people out there!" He grinned and, while Karen took the eggs and milk from the fridge, said, "The primary focus of The Power of One is your health, and that's where it first takes effect. And if you have to lose weight for your health's sake — "

"I do."

"Then you will. But if you don't, the health effects will kick in anyway. The Power of One will lower your cholesterol, your blood pressure, make you less susceptible to diabetes and heart disease and arthritis and even some cancers."

"All that?" Karen said, turning to him.

"All that and more. And when it comes to weight, there's something else I want you to keep in mind. We're not concerned with pounds. What we really want is to lower our percentage of body fat, the amount of fat our bodies have compared to all the muscle and bones and everything else. That's the real weight goal. Because even someone who thinks their weight is fine, who looks like a million bucks in their clothes, can still have too much fat in their body, while a football player, some massive bruiser who clocks in at three hundred pounds, may be, fat-wise, perfect."

"So I have to work with percentages?"

"No."

"But you said—"

"*There's no working with any numbers at all.* Not with The Power of One. In fact, you don't even have to weigh yourself."

At this Karen laughed. "I can't go without weighing myself! Especially if I'm losing weight."

"I know you can't. Neither can I. But we really don't have to—because nothing about The Power of One works with specifics. And weighing yourself every day also leaves you open to getting depressed over a weight gain that isn't even true, because our weight can move up or down a pound or two or three from one day to the next, and have nothing to do with either gaining or losing fat."

"I didn't know that," Karen said.

"It's only the bigger picture that counts. Once a week. Every two weeks. Once a month."

From the table Janice said, "When my father was losing his weight, his goal was to be down *one pound a week.* And nine out of ten weeks he did that. And continued, until he had nothing left to lose."

Karen's eyes opened wide. But Fowler shrugged aside what Janice said with a simple, "Every step in the right direction *is a success in itself,* and any progress is *exceptional progress.*" Then, stepping to the counter, he said, "I'll prepare the French toast while you make a fresh pot of tea." And, glancing back at the table, he added, "We'll also need three more glasses of water with lemon wedges."

Karen placed the kettle onto the stove and put several tea bags into the teapot, while Fowler began cracking eggs into a mixing bowl.

She watched him break open the first few eggs, then said, "What are you doing?"

"I'm preparing the eggs for the French toast."

"But the yolks...?"

One by one, Fowler was dropping the egg whites into the mixing bowl and throwing the egg yolks into the garbage, until he came to the last two eggs. Only with those did he also include the yolk. He said, "This restaurant hasn't used the same number of egg yolks as egg whites in ten years—and it never will again."

"Sometimes he saves them for other things," Janice said. "Like shampoo or conditioner or even as a repellent for his flowers."

"Waste not—want not," Fowler said.

"But won't the French toast, with only two yolks, look gross?" Karen asked.

"We'll talk about egg yolks later," Fowler said, adding, "I think a few orange slices would go well with the toast." He poured a splash of one percent milk into the eggs along with a good dash of tobasco sauce, beat the mixture well, and began to soak the bread in it. Finally he got a large nonstick frying pan from the cupboard and, after spraying it liberally with nonstick spray, started to fry the bread.

Karen poured the boiling water into the teapot, got the glasses from the table and refilled them with cold water and fresh lemon wedges, and lined up three plates, each with a couple of orange slices on it.

When the toast was golden brown on either side, Fowler put them onto the plates alongside a couple of strips of fat-reduced cheddar cheese and a hefty spoonful of fat-reduced sour cream. Then he shouted, "Pickup!" and they carried the plates to the table.

Gabe had tired of his turnip and was now testing the resiliency of Janice's cheek. Janice said, "He doesn't know what he's touching—so it doesn't bother him."

"It shouldn't bother anyone," Karen said, before taking a bite of her French toast.

Janice watched as Karen took her first bite. "How is it?"

"Excellent."

"Did you remember that there are only two egg yolks in it?"

Karen's brows rose. "No. They're—I mean, the color is perfect." She turned to Fowler.

"Karen," Fowler said, "The Power of One will solve your weight problem, I'm sure of that. But a logical way to introduce you to it, before going into details like bread or egg yolks, is to first tell you *why* you're overweight."

Karen, digging heartily into her food, laughed. "Why I'm overweight? This is why I'm overweight! Because of my appetite."

"Really...?" Fowler said. "Tell me, what would you do if Gabe didn't want to eat?"

"Well, I'd worry."

"Right. And if it persisted?"

"I'd take him to the doctor."

"Exactly. And that's because having no appetite is a sign of poor health, while having a strong appetite is a sign of good health. You're not overweight because of your appetite. No one is."

"Then what is it?"

Fowler said to Janice, "Go ahead. This is your field."

"The reason most people are overweight," Janice said, putting down her fork, "is because our bodies were designed for the way life was tens of thousands of years ago, and not today. Designed for a time when people had to search for their food. Gather it or hunt it or raise their own. Then cook it themselves. A time when individuals or small groups were in control of what they ate, because that's all there was— and they ate to stay healthy."

"You mean our food is too easy to get?" Karen asked.

"No," Janice said. "That's not it. The problem is that we've given control over our food to our modern culture. And, unlike our ancestors, our modern culture, for the most part, does not create food to keep us healthy — it creates food to make a profit."

"It helps if you realize that there are two very different groups of people involved in producing the food we eat," Fowler said. "First, there are the people who raise it for us, the farmers and ranchers and fishermen who give us all our fresh foods, all the meats and poultry and fish and vegetables and fruits and cereals. And they're the wonders of the world! God bless them all. They're our link to our ancestors, to that culture our bodies were designed for.

"And then there are the people who take that wonderful food and flip it around into burgers and fries and chips and anything else you can think of. I'm talking about the fast-food chains and the family-style restaurants and the snack-food companies and the convenience-food giants."

Janice said, "Don't leave out the cola monsters."

"You can't," Fowler said. "They and all the others are in our faces, no matter where we are. At home, out there, in our cars. And *that's* the problem. It's that they, our cultural food producers, have become so ingrained in our lives that they *are* our lives. We don't know where we end and the food giants begin. They're in our kitchens, in our cupboards, in our fridges. They're on the street, in the malls, in our grocery stores and convenience stores and drugstores and gas stations. They're everywhere. They are us. And they've twisted our minds and our children's minds into thinking that that's all there is. That what they have to offer is all there is. But it isn't."

He paused for a moment, before saying, "Think of it this way. All the parenting magazines say we should give our young children a semblance of independence, by offering them choices. For instance, the choice of what to wear. But it's still the parent who lays out the choices. The child's independence is only surface, whether to wear the blue sweater or the red sweater, because for the parent, either sweater is okay. And it's the same with the food giants. We think we have a choice, one or the other or the next. But we don't. Because beneath the surface, they're all the same. All their food is the same."

"But what else is there?" Karen asked. "They *are* everywhere. And that makes them convenient. Fast and cheap and tasty. And convenient."

"You're right," Fowler replied. "They're all of that. And you can put me at the top of the list of people who love them. Love that kind of food. And I eat it. Regularly. But I've turned the tables on them. With The Power of One I'm in control, not them. I'm the boss."

"You have the willpower to say no," Karen said.

Fowler shook his head. "If I was able to fit my willpower into a thimble, there'd still be room left over for my thumb. No. That's not it."

Janice said, "No one's willpower is strong enough to resist the pull of those food giants, because getting you to eat their products is a multi-billion-dollar business in itself. They've got the greatest scientists and sharpest advertising minds money can buy. And together they study us down to our genetic, primal urges. They know exactly how to get to us. You can't fight that kind of bombardment with willpower."

Karen leaned back in her seat. "But that's what I've always done. Hang on for a while, resist the urge, eat my lettuce, then beat myself up for doing exactly what they want me to do. Go back to them—and fail."

"You and half the country," Fowler said.

"Then what can I do?"

"You can't passively try to resist them. And you don't want to. The food giants *are* a part of our culture. A huge part. We can't *deny* that. And they'll always be a part of our lives. What you've got to do is take away their strength. Take back control. Karen, it is a war — for our health and our *children's* health. And to fight this war, like any other, you've got to be armed and ready."

CHAPTER

12

It was just past noon when Janice opened the front door.

The first words Karen said were, "I couldn't lie to him! I just don't know what he expects of me. The way he's been lately, he practically forces me to leave, then makes it worse because I come here, the only place I can go!"

Janice, with Courage at her side, said, "Come on in." Then she backed her chair deeper into the house, watchful for anyone who might be passing by. Fowler stepped up and lifted Gabe from his stroller.

Karen closed the door behind her. She could tell that Gary's refusal to allow her to become friends with Fowler and Janice disturbed them. It had affected her too, but in a different way.

Staying home, doing as Gary wished, had seemed easier than being here, effortless. And it came with the built-in rationalization that it was what Gary wanted. But even more than that, she knew, it was also that staying away from The Power of One, not learning what Fowler knew, not failing at another diet, no matter what Fowler called it, seemed easier.

But she'd told herself, No. She was going to continue through the door they'd opened, continue pushing forward with The Power of One. See where it, and they, would take her.

Fowler motioned Karen and Janice to the kitchen.

The moment Janice wheeled herself through the doorway, though, she turned her chair around and looked up at Karen and said, "We don't have to do this, you know. You can be here—just to be here. Try it that way. We can have lunch without talking about The Power of One."

"No," Karen said, taking from her bag the notebook Janice had given her and opening it to the first page. On it she'd written, *The first step to The Power of One is finding the courage to want to learn.*

Fowler read what she'd written. "Good," he said. "That is step one. And step two is to learn what there is to learn. And the best place to begin that is behind the counter."

Karen stepped to the food-preparation area with Fowler. Janice switched on the radio and parked herself at the table with Gabe. She had a magazine with her this time, one filled with mathematical puzzles. Courage stretched out on the floor beside her wheelchair.

Fowler poured two glasses of water, added lemon wedges to each, and, handing one to Karen, said, "I'm hungry. And what I'm in the mood for is a veal roll with spinach and cheese, and potato pancakes, and carrots and peas on the side, and, of course, a green salad."

Karen laughed. "What I usually have for lunch is a burger or a deli sandwich, or a submarine with a bag of chips and a soda. I don't have time to fuss, especially if I'm working."

"Well, let's see exactly what this so-called fuss is," Fowler replied. "And we'll also talk about your lunches at work, but that'll come later, not right away. Ready to start?"

"You bet. What do I do?"

"Hit the spuds," Fowler said. "We'll need about ten or so."

"Ten spuds, on the way," Karen answered. She took a sip of her water and went to work. In the meantime Fowler took three packages of veal from the fridge, put all twelve pieces onto a plate, and said, "When I cook, I never cook for just the meal I'm working on. Usually preparing a dinner for four, or a dinner for fourteen, takes virtually the same amount of time. And even if it does take a little longer, what I'm doing *is banking my energy.* And that's something else I'll tell you about later. Right now I want to start at the very beginning."

Karen nodded, and continued peeling the potatoes.

"Let me first say, and I'll keep saying this, that what I'm going to be teaching you is not a diet," Fowler explained. "Diets don't work. No matter if it's a protein diet or grapefruit diet or a counting whatever, kind of diet. They don't work because they're *unsustainable.* And that's because they rely on willpower, and if you're anything like me, willpower is in short supply."

"That," Karen said, "is the one thing I already know — from sad experience." And, she thought, if that's really true, then it takes away the worst pressure of a diet — concentrating on keeping up your willpower. Having your whole world turn into what *you can't eat.* Working with that stupid *diet mentality* of being "good" or "bad," of feeling anxious and guilty, always *guilty.* I hate that!

"The other thing I want to say," Fowler continued, "is that in all my explanations, even if I know the minute details of why certain things are the way they are, I won't go to that depth. I'll say only what's necessary. If you want you can get more information later, because it's easily available. But for our purposes, yours and mine, I'm sticking only to the major points, the ones that matter, because you have a life and I get tired of hearing my own voice. Okay?"

"Okay," Karen said.

"Good. Now let me begin by telling you there are three kinds of foods—carbohydrates, proteins, and fat. And our bodies were designed to *need all three.* That's what God did, not me. And he didn't give us any options either. So if anyone tells you the way to lose weight and gain health is by eating little or no carbohydrates or protein or fat, *they're wrong.* Just wrong. Always remember that when it comes to losing weight *and* gaining health, anything that doesn't sound like good com-monsense, anything that isn't *simple* sense, is usually *nonsense*. Got it?"

"Got it."

"Okay, so carbohydrates, or carbs, are everything that comes from plants."

"Like vegetables?"

"Right. Vegetables, fruits, and all the wheat and cereal products like bread and pasta. They're all carbs. And carbs are used by the body, like, well, the way my old clunker out there uses gas. It's our fuel.

"Proteins, on the other hand, are basically everything that comes from a source that at one time or another breathed, as well as from certain plants. So that's all animals, birds, and fish, and all their by-products, and legumes, seeds, and nuts."

"You mean meat and poultry, and dairy products and eggs?"

"Exactly. If you can trace the food's source back to something that used to breathe, it's most likely protein, plus those plant exceptions. And protein, if we go back to my clunker, is like me, that old car's mechanic. It does all the body's fixing and adjusting and maintaining."

Karen smiled.

"And the last type of food," Fowler said, "is fat. And fat, whether it comes from carbs or proteins, is anything that's greasy, like butter and oil and margarine and lard and shortening — and this," he said, holding up a strip of fat he'd trimmed from the veal. "And, again going back to the car, fat is like all the different doohickeys and fluids that the car needs. It keeps the whole thing running trouble-free."

Karen had finished peeling the potatoes and rinsing them. Now she made a motion to Fowler that said, What's next?

Fowler told her he prepared his potato pancakes in the food processor, and asked if she'd ever used one, adding, "If there's anything I can do to save time, I do it."

"You bet," Karen said. She reached up to an open shelf and took down a large bowl and began to cut the potatoes into workable, processable-size chunks. Then she started putting them through the machine.

Fowler, still working on the veal, had cut off any apparent fat, and was giving the meat a quick pounding between sheets of cellophane to make it thinner. For several minutes they worked side by side without speaking. Then Fowler continued his explanation. "To be healthy, we need all three types of food — carbs, proteins, and fat. But we need them in a certain proportion."

"Here we go," Karen said, rinsing the blades from the food processor. "This is where we start to count. And this is where I always —"

But Fowler cut her off curtly. "I said there'll be no counting of anything on my watch. No numbers. Not for anything. Life is complicated enough. All I want is for the basic proportions to be in your head. Because in this war, as in every other, knowledge is power. And the proportions are: mostly carbs, less protein, and much less fat."

"That's it?"

"That's it. And you'll soon see why you don't need numbers. Now write down what I'm going to tell you."

Karen quickly wiped her hands on a towel and reached for her notebook and pen.

"Okay," Fowler said, "the enemy is out there, all those cultural mega-giants. And in their own way, they're killing us. And the biggest weapon they're using to do this is *excess* fat. Not just fat, because as I said, we all need fat, but *excess* fat."

Karen wrote this down and underlined it, then looked at Fowler.

"So our first line of attack," Fowler continued, "our first major counterstrike against the enemy, *our first strategy*, is to reduce the amount of fat we eat — *to as low as possible*."

Then he shrugged and said, "And that's it. There's no counting of calories or fat grams or anything else. The number is *as low as possible.* And it's a strategy, not a law or religion. In some cases as low as possible is zero, while in others it's whatever it turns out to be—and that's just the way it is—because this is *real life* and not a diet."

"As low in fat as possible," Karen repeated. "No counting, just that." Then she said, "But how do I go about—"

"In practically every situation," Fowler said, raising his brows, "*there are only a few key ways to lower fat.* Only a handful. And they're all simple. And as we get to them, I'll show each one to you."

Janice, turning from one of her puzzles, said to Karen, "And once you know those key ways to lower fat—a*nd see how easy they are*— you'll be amazed at how fast this strategy gets absorbed into your life."

CHAPTER

13

"**T**hen we're on a hunt for fat," Karen said.

"That's exactly right," Fowler replied. "Always remember —
you're in a war, and the enemy's most dangerous weapon is *excess* fat.
Excess fat is his land mines, his tanks, his cruise missiles. And to
defeat the enemy you've got to eliminate his weapons. And so the
mission is to search and destroy all that excess fat!"

Karen's brows were still crouched in worry. "I know it seems
easy when you say it. Find the fat and get rid of it. But in practice it'll
be—"

"It'll be as easy as it sounds!" Fowler cocked his head and looked
Karen in the eyes, saying slowly, "Listen to me. In some situations
you'll be able to eliminate all the fat—without any effort. And in other
situations, you won't. It's as simple as that. You do what you can, then
move on with your life — without worry, without guilt. Just move
forward."

He went to the fridge and took out two containers of cheese, then
from the freezer took out two packages of frozen chopped spinach.
He popped the spinach into the microwave to thaw and held up the
containers of cheese. "Look, I've made a choice with the cheese. I
could have bought the kind that's high in fat or the kind that's fat-
reduced. And I chose the fat-reduced. Where's the difficulty there?"

"There was none."

"Right! And the veal was a choice too. I could have taken anything
off the shelf, but I took a meat that's low in fat. And the visible fat that
it did have, I removed. So I lowered the amount of fat even more."

"But there's still *some* fat in the meat," Karen said.

"Yes! Of course there is," Fowler answered. "We don't need or want to eliminate all fat. Remember what I said. Fat is essential to keeping our bodies running smoothly. We just want to get the proportions of fat into line. And so, since our culture has made us *awash* in fat, we fight back by doing what we can to make our meals as low in fat as possible—that's our mission. *And no matter the outcome, the mission is always a total success*—because we do what we can without any sacrifice or struggle, and then move on with our lives."

Karen said slowly, "So it's really that simple. As low in fat as possible. And there's no counting." Her voice, though, sounded doubtful. She knew that every diet she'd ever tried had always sounded this way at the beginning. Simple and infallible. And that whoever was trying to sell the diet, whether it was a friend or a professional pitchman, always sounded just like Fowler was sounding now, as though having her accept the diet was the most important thing in the world. But it did sound simple, didn't it?

Fowler, ignoring the tone in Karen's voice, said, "There's never any counting of anything. You go for as low in fat as possible, whatever that turns out to be—and move on."

"But what about the other percentages?" Karen asked, remembering how he'd said mostly carbs, less protein, and much less fat.

"That's coming," Fowler replied. "Let's get on with the meal first. You'll need to drain the liquid from the potatoes, then process three onions. Add them to the spuds with about a cup of flour, a tablespoon of baking powder, salt and pepper, and six eggs. But put the eggs in last, and let me know before you do it."

Karen dipped her head. Then, as an afterthought, saluted. Fowler returned the salute with a quick, full-bodied laugh and went back to his veal. He placed a sheet of wax paper on a nonstick baking pan and laid out the veal on the wax paper so that each piece overlapped the other by about half an inch. Then, after spicing the veal, he took the spinach from the microwave and put it into a mixing bowl. "What type of food is this?" he asked Karen.

"It's a plant," Karen said, "so it's a carb."

"Right. And the cheese that I'm adding to it?"

"That came from an animal, so it's a protein."

"She's got it," Fowler said to Janice.

"She does," Janice agreed.

Fowler spiced the cheese and spinach combination, mixed it well, then spread it in a thin layer over the veal.

Karen said, "Okay, everything's done except the eggs."

"Good," Fowler said. "Do you remember what I did with the eggs this morning?"

"I sure do. For about three minutes there you went temporarily insane and threw all the egg yolks, except for two, into the garbage."

Fowler, not looking in the least put off, said, "If I could have everyone in the country do just one thing for their health and their weight, it would be that— *throw all or most of their egg yolks in the garbage.* The egg white is the best source of protein we have, one that's amazingly versatile, but the yolk is a bright yellow ball of fat— and unless we need to add color to our eggs, it's out!"

"Search and destroy," Karen said.

"That's right. If you need one egg in a recipe where the egg won't be seen on its own, then use two egg whites. If you need four eggs, like now, use six or seven whites. And if you need your eggs to have their usual color, the way we did with this morning's French toast, or if we would have had them scrambled or in an omelet, then use only one egg yolk for three or four eggs. But the yolk, for the most part, is out. The fat is out. Got it?"

"Got it." Karen cracked six egg whites into her bowl, dropped all the yolks into the garbage, and got to work when Fowler told her to mix the combination well. Then she said, "Next?"

"Watch me," Fowler said. He gently lifted one side of the wax paper on which the veal was spread, and began to roll the veal over itself without letting the wax paper roll with it. When the roll was complete, he removed the wax paper, carefully centered the roll in the middle of the baking sheet, covered it with tin foil, and placed the baking sheet into a preheated oven. "There, I'm done. All in about fifteen minutes. And this is at least *ten* meals."

Then he took down a large nonstick frying pan, sprayed it liberally with nonstick cooking spray, and turned to Karen. He held up the can of spray and said, "What am I doing?"

"You're... eliminating oil."

"And what's that called?"

"Search and destroy!"

Fowler said, "I told you there were only a handful of key ways to search out and destroy fat, and you already know four of the best. And if you use only those, replace as many products as possible with their fat-reduced equivalents, use lean cuts of meat and poultry and remove all the apparent fat, use limited numbers of egg yolks *only* if you need your eggs to look yellow, and use only nonstick cooking spray in nonstick pans instead of oil or butter, you'll be miles ahead of where you are now. Miles!"

Karen nodded, knowing it was still too easy. But I am impressed, she thought, because I will try those ideas. And I wasn't planning on trying anything. All I wanted was to understand The Power of One.

Fowler put the frying pan on a burner, turned the heat to medium, and said, "Okay, spoon the potato mixture into the pan, and make them small — three inches at most." While Karen did this, Fowler said, "What you're going to find is that after a while, after you've been hunting and destroying fat for a few months, you'll begin to lose the taste for it."

"Lose the taste for fat?"

"Yes."

"Now that's hard to believe."

"You will. Six months from now you might go into a restaurant for breakfast and order toast and it'll come dripping with butter, when you've been using fat-reduced cream cheese or jam or marmalade all those months, and you won't like the taste of the butter. You'll see, you won't like the feel of it in your throat or on the top of your mouth. The body loses the urge for it."

"I can't believe that," Karen said.

Janice said, "I don't know why, but it's true."

"You can count on it," Fowler added. "It happened to both of us." Then he said, "Okay, back to the meal. What else was on the menu?"

Karen had already spooned eight pancakes into the pan, flattened them so they were thin, the way Fowler suggested, let them brown, flipped them over, and when they were ready, placed them on a tray. Now she spooned in eight more, saying, "The rest of the menu—peas and carrots and a green salad." Then she added, "You know, about now, if I was alone and the cooking was being done because it had to be done, and not because I was having a good time, I'd be getting pretty tired of it. Actually, by this point, I doubt if I'd want to do anything else — not peel one carrot or clean a single lettuce leaf." Then she shook her head, and in a tone that could only be called surrender, said, "It's what Gary always says. It's my lazy streak."

"There's a difference between being lazy and being tired," Fowler quickly replied," or needing a break. Or getting a hand once in a while. You're a mother and a wife and you work outside the home. And in today's world we don't have to work in the fields to get tired. Just sitting at a desk is work enough, handling our responsibilities at home and in the office and in our relationships can be more than enough. And if sometimes you do feel lazy, well, I'll raise your lazy with two of my own, because we've all got a lazy streak in us.

"So let me show you two ways to get around being tired. And if you want to call it lazy, then let's call it lazy. A very, very positive lazy.

"First," he said, going to the freezer, "here's our peas and carrots." He took out a bag of frozen peas and carrots, poured it into a pot, filled the pot with water, and put it on to boil. "There. That's done. One minute, maybe less. Now the salad." He went to the fridge, took out a bag of store-bought prewashed greens, opened the bag and dropped them into a bowl, added some fat-reduced salad dressing, and said, "There's the salad. Another minute."

Karen was smiling. You got me, she thought, finishing the last of the potato pancakes.

Fowler turned to her. "Karen," he said, "*The Power of One is real life, not playing house. Not playing diet.* Not playing at anything. If there's something out there that's nutritious and quick to prepare and fits into the strategies, then go for it! We're not here to be martyrs or masochists. Okay?"

"Okay," Karen said, adding, "How many strategies are there?"

"Only eight," Fowler answered her, opening the oven door. "That's all you need." He took out the veal, placed it next to the tray of potato pancakes, and turned to Karen again. "Watch — and learn how to blow that term *lazy* off the map!"

He took down three plates from one cupboard, then from another took out seven plastic containers. He lined the containers in a row and, after slicing the veal into ten equal portions, placed one portion into each of the containers, along with three potato pancakes and a good helping of the peas and carrots. Then he sealed the containers and said, touching each container after the other, "This is for your lunch tomorrow. And this is your dinner on Wednesday. And this one is a late-night snack in July. And this is your breakfast in early September — "

"Yuck."

"Hey, that's good food. And the last three are for whenever you want." Then he took Karen by the elbow, led her to the freezer, opened the door, and said, "And all of these, all fifteen or twenty different meals and snacks, *were made when the making was good.* When the energy level was high. Or just when I had to cook something, anything, and out of habit, made more than I needed and stored the rest here, in my energy bank, for those days or nights or mornings when the only thing on my mind is to throw something into the microwave and drop my butt into a chair."

Janice said, "I don't think you can call someone who'd prepared for their tired times lazy. A better word might be *ingenious.*"

Fowler, seeming to take no notice of Janice's compliment, said, "Okay, now you know that the first strategy of The Power of One is to eat as little fat as possible — by making thoughtful choices — without letting the strategy intrude into your life. *Without any sacrifice or struggle, without feeling anxious or guilty.* But there was one more item in this strategy that we touched on, but didn't finish. The proportions."

"That's right," Karen said. "The proportions of carbs to protein to fat." Then she said, "Mostly carbs, less protein, and much less fat. But how do I make sure?"

"Watch," Fowler replied. He put the remaining three portions of veal onto the three plates. Then to each he added three potato pancakes, a good serving of the peas and carrots, and a hefty portion of the salad. "Now," he said. "If you look at what we have in our plates, you'll see that a small part of the plate has the veal and cheese..."

"The protein," Karen said.

"Right. And a much larger part of the plate has the potatoes and carrots and peas and the salad."

"The carbs."

"Right. And it's as simple as that. Because those are the proportions we're used to. Mostly carbs, less protein..."

"And the fat," Karen said, "because of the strategy of search and destroy, of making it as low in fat as possible, is also where it's supposed to be, in proportion. And there was no counting of anything."

Fowler nodded. "If we take care of the fat, the rest will take care of itself. And remember too that those basic percentages the body needs are important for the big picture, a twelve or twenty-four-hour period. They aren't necessary for every meal or every snack. So just because you know about them doesn't mean you even have to think about them."

"Except for the fat," Karen said.

Fowler grinned. "That's what the strategy says—and that's all you have to remember."

In a tone filled with surprise, Karen said, "It is simple, isn't it?"

CHAPTER

14

For the next three days Karen worked, so there was no opportunity to visit Janice and Fowler. Then she spent a quiet weekend with Gabe while Gary watched sports on television. During this time his only mention of Janice and Fowler was a quick aside about "those nuts in the woods."

She telephoned them, though, and was overjoyed to find that they were as happy to hear from her as she was to speak to them. She arranged to go to their house first thing Monday, and the moment Gary left for work that morning she bundled Gabe into his stroller.

She hadn't done anything about The Power of One during the past five days except think about it. Go over and over in her mind the few things Fowler had so far explained. Now she whispered, "I'm an idiot," and thought, What he's told me so far is ridiculously simple. There's not even any effort involved. *It's all just a matter of choices.* And I still haven't been able to start it. Then she thought, A pound a week, that's all he wants. Week after week. Month after month.

Suddenly she said to herself, Wait a minute! What I'm doing is filling my brain with doubts by looking at *that* end of it, at how *long* it's going to take, when I ought to be looking at it from *this* side. The now. *Today*. Looking at the first step Fowler talked about. Looking only at that. I'm basing beginning The Power of One on what I don't know, instead of what *I do know*!

Then she thought, *Today*. That's the key! Small steps—and today. Now! But with this thought she winced, feeling the old familiar mix of fear and dread rise up from the knot in her gut, and her next thought was, Courage. It always keeps coming back to that. That tiny amount of courage, that *first step* courage. The courage I need to get me to do what has to be done — today. Without thinking about tomorrow. And then tomorrow will just be another today. And all of it without the old diet attitude, diet mentality.

She stopped walking, reached into her bag, and took out her notebook. Kneeling on the sidewalk next to Gabe, she wrote: *The enemy is out there and he's making me fat. It's not my fault — no matter what Gary thinks! But I can defeat the enemy. Fowler's proven that by doing it. And the weapons I need to defeat the enemy are courage and knowledge.*

She read this through and underlined *courage* and *knowledge*, then wrote: *Knowledge can be learned, I see that now. There's nothing difficult about what Fowler's telling me. But courage, that's something else altogether. I don't know where courage comes from. I never have.*

Janice greeted Karen with another wonderful welcome, saying, "Why don't we go into the den until my father wakes up, so we can talk without disturbing him."

She led the way, closing the door after Karen, motioning her to an easy chair alongside one of the desks where the computer was switched on. "I was working," she said, stopping her chair in front of the desk. She reached out to touch Gabe, who was content this morning to sit quietly in Karen's lap.

"He had the sniffles most of the night, poor thing," Karen said, "so he'll probably spend the day catching up on his sleep." She comforted Gabe, adjusting him in her arms, then looked at the computer screen. It was filled with text. She began to read the first line, bumping into the words *monocultures, biodiversity,* and *transgenic.*

Janice said, "I'm part of a team based in the U.K. that's refuting the government's claim about the safety of genetically modified foods."

"The U.K.?"

Janice nodded. "I do a lot of work over the internet."

"Is this your job?" Karen asked, looking at the screen once more.

"No. It's a nonprofit group, so there's no salary. But I'm glad to do it. I have been offered a position with another think tank, though — actually several — but of course it's impossible for me to work."

"Why?"

For a moment Janice only stared at Karen. Then she said, "Because I can't leave this house, can't let myself be seen. Because people are... shocked." She paused for a moment, then in a lowered voice added, "I can only imagine how my father felt when he first saw me. And my mother..." She let the word mother fade, before saying, "For a long time it was hard on him, having to deal with someone like me, a one-in-a-million mistake with complication after complication."

Karen reached out and touched Janice's hand, holding it for a moment without speaking.

"Fortunately things changed," Janice said, her voice resuming its usual tone.

"Changed?" Karen said. "Because of The Power of One?"

Janice nodded. "It's impossible to tell you how much The Power of One turned my father's life around, and because of that, mine."

Karen thought of the bottle of whisky on the wall of Fowler's restaurant, and the pair of trousers mounted like a trophy, and realized they represented the most significant successes of Fowler's life. He found The Power of One, she thought, opened its door, and he and Janice stepped through it into a new world. She found herself wishing, If only the same could happen to me and Gary. Then she said to Janice, "Tell me about your father."

Janice began by saying, "I love him." Then, "Just like everyone else, he had his problems — he still does. And one of those problems is me, I guess. And at first he handled those problems the way a lot of people do, by using crutches—food, alcohol, cigarettes—to get him through the day. Using that to comfort himself. And like a lot of people, he didn't notice or care what he was doing until those escapes became his real problems. Took over his life. When he first decided to do something about it, he weighed over three hundred pounds."

"But how did he start? I mean... What was...? What did...?" She searched for the right word.

Janice said, "What was the spark, besides his mirror?"

But before she could answer her own question, the door opened and Fowler, sleep still in his eyes, peeked into the room. "I saw the stroller in the hall," he said. "Good morning."

"I guess he can tell you what the spark was himself," Janice said to Karen. Then she turned to Fowler. "Karen wants to know what spark, besides your mirror, got you to develop The Power of One."

Fowler stepped into the room. "The spark wasn't my mirror. All the mirror did was make me feel guilty and weak."

"Then what was the spark?" Karen asked.

"The spark was anger. I was angry. Furious! At me. At my size. At my food. At my mirror. At all of it. And I used that anger to begin my journey."

"To begin The Power of One?" Karen said.

"Eventually. But only after a thousand attempts, after a hundred useless diets that limit what you eat, or put you on pills or liquids or only proteins, all of them tied to willpower, all designed to make you lose thirty pounds in thirty days, so you can gain back thirty-five a month later." He grinned.

Karen's expression, though, was somber. "I know you keep saying The Power of One isn't a diet. But if it's not a diet, then what is it?"

"I've thought about that," Janice said, "and I think what it is is a map."

"A map?"

"Yes. A nutritional road map. Pointing the way from here to the city of Health." She paused, then added, "But it's even more than that. *It's a new way of thinking.* It's tomorrow, beginning now. In five or ten or twenty years, The Power of One will be the nutritional road map the nation will be using—because it's not only based on science, but also on *real life and good commonsense.* People won't let The Enemy win this war—because they can't afford to, for their health's sake. So they'll ultimately dictate the way things are going to be, for themselves and their children, and not the other way around, the way it is now."

Karen was nodding her head, not only thinking about what Janice just said, but also about the entry she'd made in her journal this morning. She asked, "If the first step into The Power of One is just a tiny amount of courage, just enough to say to myself that I really want to lose weight and that I'll make the simple choices at hand, then why is it that even that *small* amount is so hard for me to find?"

Fowler, after reflecting on the question, said, "I think the short answer is fear. You're afraid. And you're afraid of two things. First, you're afraid of having to give up the foods you've grown to depend on. Your *comfort foods.* Whether it's ice cream or chocolate or pizza or anything else. Those foods have become extremely important to you, to your life.

"And second, it's the old fear of failure. And those two fears work hand in hand."

"How?" Karen wanted to know.

"Over the years," Fowler said, "we've been swayed by everything from word of mouth to slick, hour-long infomercials playing on our sense of guilt or shame, into trying too many wonder diets, too many magic pills. And all we got for our efforts—our sincere efforts—was failure. Not only did we have to give up what we liked, and even needed—those comfort foods we'd grown up with—but we were also forced into complicated programs of calorie counts or fat gram counts or trying to keep straight in our heads or in little booklets which food we were allowed to eat with which other food and on what day and at what time of day. And on and on and on.

"And in time all that nonsense and intrusion into our real, everyday lives became too much, inevitably so, so we ultimately ended it — ended the diet—ended it in failure, even if we'd lost some weight— *because diets are not sustainable.*

"And that made our only frame of reference when it came to losing weight, to dieting, failure. And it was that reference we carried with us to our next attempt. But by now our minds were saying, No! I won't put myself through *that* again. The struggle's too hard. Too painful. And not worth it. I won't set myself up for another failure!

"Or else we did give it another try, did get lured into another irresistibly slick wonder diet. But by now the attempt was half-hearted, no matter what we said, even to ourselves. It was half-hearted on the inside, where it counts, because by now *we knew we were going to fail. We were living with the diet mentality of pain and guilt and failure.* We expected failure and so we did fail. And still do. Always. I know the cycle. I lived it over and over and over."

Janice, turning to Karen, said, "Is that what your mind is telling you? Now? About The Power of One?"

Karen nodded.

Fowler said, "Even though you know that The Power of One is not a diet? That its strategies *accommodate* life, become a *part* of it, do not *interfere* with it? And even though you know there's no such thing as a food you aren't allowed to eat?"

Karen nodded again, then, in a resigned tone, said, "Somehow it doesn't matter how you describe it. In my mind The Power of One is still a diet, and I still need courage to attempt it. You were exactly right when you said my lack of courage comes from fear. And exhaustion. From that diet mentality. I'm tired of failing and my mind is screaming at me that I will fail again. That I'm only going to disappoint myself, and disappoint you, and, for the thousandth time, confirm Gary's opinion of me."

"I know what you're feeling," Fowler said, "because I've been there. So I also know it's useless for me to try to talk you into changing those feelings. So I won't."

"You won't?" Karen said, suddenly disappointed. She turned to Janice, who also looked let down.

Fowler shook his head no. Then, grinning, he said, "What I will do is prove to you, right now, that The Power of One is different. That it's not a diet. That there's no struggling with it. And that it can so completely fit into your life, you won't even know it's there."

He waited a moment before saying, "What did you do with the seven meals I gave you the last time you were here?"

Karen smiled sheepishly. "I ate them."

"When did you eat them?"

"I ate the first two on the same day you gave them to me. One for dinner, then the other after Gary went to bed."

Fowler said, "That's good."

"But I ate the same meal three times in one day, once for lunch with you, then again for dinner, then again for a late-night snack."

"So what? Your body doesn't care about that. All your body wants is for the meals you eat to be nutritious. Which they were. When did you eat the rest?"

"You're going to laugh at me," Karen said.

Fowler's expression told her differently.

"I ate another for lunch at work the next day, warming it in their microwave. Then I had another for dinner, before Gary got home. Then again I had another after he went to bed, around ten-thirty."

"Excellent!"

"You mean it?"

"Of course! You had three nutritious, lower-in-fat-than-usual, meals in one day. That's great. What about the rest?"

"Gary ate them. I just heated them together and put them in a plate and told him it was from the deli, and he wolfed them down."

Fowler laughed. "Okay. Now I'm going to make my point. Prove that you *can't fail* with The Power of One." He paused, looked Karen in the eyes, then said, "No matter what else you did last week, you already broke The Enemy's grip on you—because you had five meals that were nutritionally perfect. You struck perfection *five* times. With that, you took your first step! Had your first success. Advanced your health. You did it, Karen. You met the goal of The Power of One!"

It took a moment for Karen to fully grasp what Fowler had just said. Then, with a wondering smile spreading across her lips, she whispered, "I have advanced my health, haven't I?"

"Yes!"

"And advancing my health is the goal of The Power of One?"

"Yes!"

"And part of advancing my health is losing weight?"

"Yes!"

Karen's eyes were wide, alight. "And it was because of those five meals. That's all it took. They were the first step I was looking for and I took it without even knowing it."

"That's the way The Power of One is *designed* to work," Fowler said. "It *disappears into your life*, instead of being an intrusion upon it." He grinned. "What are you feeling now? At this exact moment?"

"I'm feeling that I want to eat more of those meals! Push myself even further ahead."

"Further ahead? Keep meeting the goal? Keep acquiring successes? Keep gaining health and losing weight?"

"Yes!"

"Well, that feeling is not accidental. That's the *momentum* created by The Power of One. When you see how simple it is to know, for sure, that you've achieved a degree of health, then you want to push yourself even further."

"But it was so easy," Karen said. "Almost *too* easy. All I did was eat."

"*All you did was adjust to the circumstances at hand, and not fall into the 'all or nothing' trap of the diet mentality*. Those meals were there and you ate them. The Power of One *slipped* into your life. And remember, all you know of The Power of One so far is the first strategy. And even with that strategy, you still don't know all I'm going to teach you. Imagine when you have all the knowledge inside you. Imagine having an *infinite number of combinations* to work with, to adjust to your own circumstances."

"I'll be able to use what I want of it then," Karen said. "Let it adjust to me. Fit me."

"Exactly. That's why you can't fail. Because once the knowledge is in you, once you understand the strategies, then you can tailor The Power of One to *suit your life at every moment*, no matter the situation. And then readjust it. And you'll still, always, be moving toward the goal."

"My goal is to lose weight."

"No!" Fowler said adamantly. "Your goal is to gain health — only that — incrementally and continuously, *for the rest of your life*. If your weight is a health problem, then your weight *will* be reduced."

Karen said, "It's that focus too that makes it different, sort of puts it into a different light. The Power of One is not just for overweight people, it's for everyone."

"That's right. The Power of One is not a diet — and it's not specifically for overweight people. It's for *anyone who cares about his or hers or their children's health.*"

CHAPTER

15

"**I** want to learn more!" Karen said.

Janice, reaching for her computer keyboard, said, "I've still got a good hour's work here." Then she looked at Gabe and said softly, "He's fast asleep."

"Why don't we go into the restaurant and have a coffee and talk," Fowler said to Karen, "and when Janice is ready, we'll cook a Power of One breakfast." He stood, mouthing the word *coffee*? to Janice.

Janice nodded yes, then said to Karen, "Can Gabe sleep in here? I'll keep an eye on him for you."

At the table, after Fowler had made coffee and brought one to Janice, Karen said, "You gave me four simple ways to reduce fat, but a few minutes ago you said there was still more to the first strategy."

"That's right," Fowler answered. He was quickly sifting through the mail, which had just arrived. He put the small pile of letters and magazines down on the table and turned to Karen. "Okay, there's a basic rule to keep in mind about fat, and that is that *fat is almost everywhere*. So our first job is to *find* the fat. Because you can only get rid of it, as much as possible, after you've found it." He smiled, then said playfully, "Why don't we think of finding fat... in terms of a party?"

"A party? I thought we were fighting a war."

Now he laughed. "We are fighting a war! But at the moment we're not just ordinary soldiers, we're highly trained spies. We're James Bond."

Karen raised her brows. "James Bond and Jane Bond!"

"Right! James and Jane. And we're at this party in..."

"Tangier!"

"That's it. Now you're getting it. Can you feel the intrigue? The undercurrent of powerful forces?"

"Good versus evil."

"Exactly. Good versus evil. And we're the good guys."

"Of course."

"And the bad guys are...?"

"Fat!"

"Right! Fat! But they're devious, those bad fats, because they're trying to..."

"Seduce us!"

"That's it! They want to seduce us. But they can't unless we let them, because we know who they are. They're the noisiest, brashest, most exciting people at the party. They're uninhibited, dance to the most intense beats, laugh the loudest."

"They're the most fun to be with!"

"That they are," Fowler replied. "But...?"

"But? But what?"

"Come on, Jane Bond. Work with me."

Karen said, "But we're too smart for them?"

"That's right. We are too smart for them. But how are we too smart for them?"

"We're too smart for them because we know what they want."

"Exactly! And what do they want?"

"They want us to take them home so they can get under our skin and live on our hips."

"Right!" Fowler said. "But we won't let that happen, because now that we know who they are, we're going to do our job, do what we're trained for—we're going to take them out!"

"Search and destroy!"

"That's it! And we'll begin by leaving those bad fats at the party and taking home only the good guys."

"Our guys."

"Yes! Our guys. And bringing them into a safe, *defatted* haven."

"A what?" Karen asked.

Fowler swept his hand toward the cooking area. "A safe, defatted haven. Please, Jane, won't you follow me into my haven and let me show you what you don't see." He stood and Karen followed him around the counter to the refrigerator. Fowler opened the door. "Okay, what don't you see?"

Karen looked in, waited a sincere moment, then said, "How can I know what I don't see?"

"The first thing you don't see," Fowler said, "is butter."

"That's right, there's no butter."

"Now, what *do* you see?"

Karen laughed lightly, realizing where Fowler was going. "I see fat-reduced cream cheese, fat-reduced mayonnaise. Other cheeses that are fat-reduced. One percent milk. And I'm beginning to see what you mean."

"Of course you see what I mean. The only full fat I allow in this fat-reduced haven is a small bottle of very good olive oil, because there are times when I like very good olive oil. And for me, that's it. Those are the conditions I want here, in my haven. This, for now, is the degree to which I want the first strategy tailored to *my* home and *my* life. The degree I brought it to after deciding, food item by food item, what would work *for me*. Because The Power of One is not a diet."

He grinned. "You see, I don't have to accommodate it, it has to accommodate me. Here, in my home, The Power of One accommodates me. And outside of here, in that other world, The Power of One still accommodates me, because there I adjust its strategies to fit those changed circumstances, even circumstances that are out of my control."

Karen said, "So just because a circumstance may be out of your hands, The Power of One never is. You always have control, in every situation, because you control The Power of One."

"Exactly. I understand the strategies and that allows me to control them, *tailor them to my needs...* It becomes clearer when you keep reminding yourself of the basics. And what are the basics?"

For a moment Karen looked puzzled, then she said slowly, "That The Power of One is not a diet."

"Right. That's key. It's not a diet. It's not designed to reach a specific number then come to an end. What else?"

"That every element of it is flexible."

Fowler nodded. "That gives it its adaptability. The quality to fit your life at every moment of your life. And next?" he said. "The big one? The big picture?"

Karen thought, but was stumped.

Fowler said to her, "This one I'm going to keep telling you until you see it in your dreams, because this is what we want out of The Power of One every day. Every single day."

"Then wait a second," Karen said. She went back to the table, got her notebook and pen, and returned. "Okay, say it slowly, so I can write it down."

Fowler said, *"The goal of The Power of One is to gain health through nutrition—always that—incrementally and continuously, for the rest of our lives.* And every step, every tiny step toward that goal, *is a success in itself.*"

Karen wrote the words he'd just told her, then said, "That is all you want, isn't it? For me to just move in the right direction. Using those small steps. Those easy steps. Steps that can be continually adjusted to fit my life no matter the situation."

Fowler dipped his head and Karen said, "It is a journey. An almost pleasant stroll. One step, then another. One success, then another. Use a piece of this strategy, a piece of that. Smell the flowers. Take a step. Smile at the neighbors. Take a step. No great sacrifice. No numbers to meet. Nothing to count. Just the step. That's the goal! Take a step, meet your goal. Hello, goal."

She laughed and said, "And I've already begun! And it was so simple I didn't even realize it! There was no waiting for the right day, no counting down the minutes until I had to go on it. No stuffing my face with all the usual junk, knowing I wouldn't be able to have that great-tasting garbage again until this diet also fails. The five meals I ate were delicious and the first small steps in the right direction. The first successes. I'm already headed toward nutritional health and losing weight."

She laughed again. "Take a step. Then another. For the rest of my life. That's all there is to it. And the first step will lead to the next. And that'll lead to another. And it'll all lead to excitement — the excitement I'm feeling now. And it's that excitement that'll push me forward!"

But even as Fowler was agreeing with her, she thought, This might have worked for you. But it's not going to work for me. And she said, "I'm sorry, Fowler. I can't... I mean, no matter what you say, I still don't think I'll, you know, succeed." She shrugged her shoulders and again whispered, "Sorry."

But Fowler, suddenly animated, said, "Perfect! That's perfect! That's the definition of healthy skepticism I was waiting for. Now you're beginning to remind me of me!" Then he said, "Okay, we're rolling here, and it's time for me to tell you about creativity."

Karen, wearing a wondering smile, said, "Creativity? Is that one of the strategies?"

"No. But it's just as important. Let me put it to you this way — what I'm seeing is our platoon."

"Platoon? We're back to the war?"

"Always! Never forget that. This is a constant battle, no matter how invisible it becomes. We're fighting those forces out there for our family's health and our own! And our platoon is armed with eight strategies, and those strategies are so strong, so powerful, that we know with just them, we can take on The Enemy. But we have even more than the eight strategies to rely on. We have surrounding us two more layers of protection and those layers are defensive, not offensive. And one of them is the courage that you already know about, that tiny amount of necessary courage. And the other, within our defensive ring of courage, is creativity. Are you following so far?"

"Yes. And I like it," Karen said, consciously deciding to ignore her doubts and just follow wherever Fowler led. "I'm going to be armed with eight strategies and protected even more by a ring of courage and, within that ring, an inner ring of creativity. And I know about courage. I know that I don't need much of it, just the tiny amount *I'm using now to learn what there is to learn*. But what do you mean by creativity?"

"Creativity is just that, being creative. And we've already talked about it. We just didn't define it. But creativity is so important to The Power of One that it's got to be defined."

"When did we talk about it?"

"We talked about it when we talked about ways of getting rid of fat. Eliminating egg yolks is creative. Replacing cooking oil with nonstick pans and sprays is creative."

"And," Karen said, "eating the meals you gave me to take home, three times in one day, is really creative."

"That's right. Because for us, creativity, when you get right down to it, *is the way in which we tailor each of The Power of One's strategies to suit ourselves.*"

"So what you're saying, then," Karen said, "is that creativity is the quality that gives The Power of One its flexibility. It's infinite flexibility."

"That's exactly right. The only hard rule in The Power of One is that there are *no hard rules.* The strategies, tucked inside courage, can be shaped and molded by creativity to fit your needs at every moment."

"But what if I haven't got a creative bone in my body. Which I don't."

"Then you'll still use creativity, but you'll just call it by another name, like *wiggle room or how about this, instead of that, or let me test this strategy one degree at a time.* And then there's my old favorite, *that's good enough for today, because it was better than yesterday.*"

Fowler grinned. "The point I want to make is that all through The Power of One, creativity, by whatever name, comes into play with every strategy. And it's important to keep creativity's flexibility in mind."

"Courage, to get the war started," Karen said. "Creativity to keep it personally tailored and infinitely mobile, and the strategies themselves to wallop The Enemy."

"You got it."

CHAPTER

16

Courage padded into the room, walked around the counter to Fowler, and nudged his hand.

Fowler said, "Nature's calling," and smiled. He began to turn to the door, then said to Karen, "Why don't we go out with him, for a short walk in the garden?"

"I'd love to walk through the garden," Karen said. "All I've seen of it so far is the view from the window. I'll just go see how Gabe's doing."

Fowler was on the porch when Karen stepped outside. He handed her an orange, and started peeling one of his own.

Karen, standing at the porch railing that overlooked the lawn, said, "It's stunning."

"It's been a thirty-year labor of love," Fowler replied. "The farm itself is close to thirty acres, most of it fields, none of it in cultivation. But the garden, well, it's closing in on four acres now, and that's about as much as any one person can handle."

"It must be a huge job," Karen said.

"From March to October it doesn't let you take much time off, but no, the way it's designed, a lot of it takes care of itself." He motioned Karen down the stairs and to a cobblestone walk that arced toward a spectacular weeping willow. "These borders, for example. They're designed to be easily cut with one pass of a riding mower. Made so I can get right up to the perennial beds without slowing down. There's no fussiness about it, not like some of your city gardens."

Karen was taking in the spectacular view.

Handing her a section of his orange, Fowler said, "I like to look at the garden the same way I look at The Power of One. It's got to fit in. Fit me. No element of it can take up more of my time than I think that element's worth, otherwise it begins to gnaw at my nerves." He finished eating the orange in his hand, then asked Karen for hers, and began peeling that one too.

Karen said, "I never realized that making something disappear into your life could take so much forethought. Planning."

"Now you're talking about The Power of One," Fowler said.

"Lately that's all I think about—The Power of One, and food. But never in the way you do."

"Tell me about that," Fowler said, turning to her. "Tell me how you start your food day."

"You mean breakfast?"

Fowler nodded. "Breakfast on a workday."

"There is no breakfast on a workday. It's impossible. First there's Gary. Getting him out of the house. Taking care of whatever he needs. And Gabe. Preparing him for the sitter, then dropping him off at her house, then driving into town and hopefully getting to the office by nine."

"So when is the first time you eat in the morning?" Fowler asked.

"About ten, ten-fifteen. That's when I get a donut and coffee from the snack bar in the building."

Courage ran across an open section of lawn. Fowler laughed. "He likes to lord it over the squirrels, tell 'em who's boss." Then, facing Karen again, he said, "We talked about creativity, so now I want you to work with me to find your creative streak."

Karen nodded.

"If you wanted," Fowler continued, "could you have your donut and coffee earlier?"

Without hesitation Karen replied, "Sure. I could have it as soon as I walk into the office. Just pick it up on the way in and eat it at my desk like everyone else. Except that that early in the morning, I'm not hungry." Then, with a shrug, she said, "Actually, it's not so much that I'm not hungry. It's more that first thing in the morning I don't feel like I have to eat. And let's face it, the less I eat, the better. So I don't. I just wait — and hope that one day all that waiting will add up to the loss of a pound or two."

Fowler handed her another orange section. "I'll let you in on a little secret. It's impossible to lose weight by skipping breakfast. In fact, skipping breakfast has the opposite effect. *Skipping breakfast contributes to weight gain, while eating breakfast contributes to weight loss.*"

"What?" Karen said, stopping and looking at Fowler. "That doesn't sound right. How can not eating contribute to gaining weight?"

Fowler divided the last of the orange sections, gave Karen half, and said, *"Strategy Number Two. You have to eat breakfast."*

"But why? I don't understand."

"Well, it's like this. Apart from anything you might think, a large part of the work our bodies do in a twenty-four-hour period is digest our food, break down the carbs and proteins and fats we eat into the nutrients our bodies need. And it does this work during the day, during our eating hours, then continues this work at night."

He paused. "Maybe I can explain it this way. Remember I said that the carbs we eat are used by the body as fuel?"

"Sure. You were talking about your car. And the proteins are used as the mechanics and the fat is like all the different additives we put in to keep everything running smoothly."

"Right. For our purposes, that's exactly right. And throughout the day we feed those basic food elements to our body and it uses what it needs during the day, and also uses what it needs at night."

"The car's night crew."

"Exactly. The night crew. And the day crew and night crew are hardworking guys who sweat away at their jobs, fueling and maintaining and adding important parts. And while they sweat, you're burning calories, and, if other conditions are right, if your strategies are up and running, *that burning of calories means you're losing weight.* But by the time early morning comes around, the night crew's shift is over, and they go home. The day crew, though, can't get in until you eat breakfast, so they're left standing on the sidewalk."

Karen was trying to picture all this in her mind.

"Breakfast," Fowler continued, "is the key that opens the door for the day crew. Without it, all they can do is stand around and shuffle their feet and wait. So the car, your body, without any fuel, without any mechanics, is basically shut down. Oh sure, the light for the alarm still blinks and the clock still works. You can breathe and talk and take care of Gabe. But the essentials on the inside are at a standstill. The car is parked. It's sitting in the garage. And none of the really important work gets done because you're not burning *enough* calories, and without that, you're not losing weight. Breakfast lets the day crew crank the ignition and press down hard on the gas. It starts your engine. Gets everything working again."

Karen stopped and stared at Fowler. "So what you're saying is that I have to eat to lose weight?"

"Yes! Of course you have to eat! Eating is not what's making you fat. The Enemy is making you fat!" Fowler shook his head. "To lose weight consistently, sustainably, and in a way that you're also gaining health, you have to eat."

"Okay," Karen said. "Let me get this straight. If it's not eating that's making me fat, then it's what they, The Enemy, are giving me to eat, advertising me into eating. And if I just follow the strategies..."

"You now know two strategies. And if you use just those two, to the degree that fits your circumstances, you'll lose weight. Without a doubt, you'll lose weight. But losing weight is not the point."

"No," Karen answered, still thinking about what Fowler just said. "Losing weight is not the point. The point is gaining health. But," she added, "losing weight would be so, so..."

"Exciting?" Fowler asked.

"You'd better believe it!"

"I do believe it. In fact, I still feel it every day, every morning when I weigh myself, every morning when I walk into the restaurant and see those trousers on the wall." He smiled. "Okay, let's go through it again, just to make sure you got it right, but this time you do it."

Karen's eyes were shining. She said, "Strategy number two — I have to eat breakfast. And with my new creative streak, I can pick it up on the way in to the office and eat it at nine o'clock, easily."

"Eat what?" Fowler asked.

"Eat my..." She paused, thought for a moment, then said, laughing, "Eat my fried-in-lard, filled-with-fat donut. Or else I could order a bagel, or toast, spread with jam, or fat-reduced cream cheese."

"That's it!" Fowler replied. "Make the bagel whole wheat or the bread multigrain."

"Or," Karen said, her words racing, "I can have an orange like now or a banana or even one of your delicious meals meant for supper."

"Now we're talking strategies!" Fowler said, motioning toward another path, this one veering back toward the house.

Karen, shaking her head, said, "You know, what we're talking about is so simple. Breakfast on workdays. Just that. No big deal. Just something quick and easy to put into my mouth. And the lower-fat choices are there. They're easily available..."

"That's something else I wanted to hear," Fowler said. "It's not a big deal. Let's not obsess over a single breakfast, or snack, or meal. Let's not obsess over anything to do with eating. It's just eating. There's always the next meal, and it's there the moment you want it."

"You're right," Karen said. "I know you're right. But do you want to know something? At this moment I am looking forward to that workday breakfast — just so I can know I'm following the first two strategies perfectly — for that meal, at least. And it's going to be easy."

They crested a small hill, then stepped through a funnel of box hedge that opened onto a large crescent-shaped lily pond. Courage was on the other side of the pond.

"Every bend of this path exposes another world," Karen said. "And each looks as though it's been here for a thousand years."

"I like to have the garden blend into the landscape," Fowler replied, "until the landscape begins to flow from the garden. They become one — the garden, the distant trees, the sky. There can be no lines, no breaks."

"The Power of One," Karen said.

Fowler grinned. "The similarity is not accidental."

CHAPTER

17

"**O**kay," Fowler said, while they were heading back to the house. "Tell me what you usually eat for breakfast on the days you don't work."

"Well," Karen replied. "Two of the days I don't work are still weekdays, not long, lazy Sunday mornings, so I still have to have something quick and easy."

"Okay," Fowler said. "We're talking about Monday and Tuesday and Saturday mornings too."

Karen nodded. "You can also add Sundays to that list. I can't even remember the last time I had a lazy morning in bed." Then she quickly added, "I guess what I'd usually have, if I have anything more than a coffee, is a bowl of sugar coated pops or a pop-in-the-toaster-tart or two." She laughed at the sudden, exaggerated look of shock on Fowler's face, then asked, "What happened? What did I say?"

"What you said," Fowler answered, "was the cue for me to give you *strategy number three. Eat as little sugar as possible.*"

For a moment Karen only looked at Fowler. Then, shaking her head, she said, "Here it is. Here, for me, is where The Power of One falls apart."

"It won't."

"It will! You just don't know. My sweet tooth is the size of Connecticut."

"And mine is the size of Texas," Fowler said.

"So what do you do?"

"I accommodate it. Within the flexibility of the strategies."

"How?"

"I'll tell you how. But first I want to tell you why. And it goes like this. Although sugar is a carb, *it's an empty carb, a simple carb filled with useless calories.* And if we go back to my old clunker..."

"Where carbs are the fuel," Karen said.

"Right. Where carbs are the fuel, then sugar carbs are the exception. They're the only carbs that don't work. Putting them into the car is like putting in sewage. You can fill up the tank with it, turn the key in the ignition, and press down on the gas — but the only thing that'll happen is the car will sputter and stall and get uselessly fat! What you end up with is a mess."

"That's me," Karen said.

"And," Fowler continued, "just like fat, sugar is also a master of disguise, coming in all shapes and colors and sizes. Also trying to find its way into your life."

"And onto my second chin," Karen added.

"It sounds like you've met sugar before."

"Have I ever. He's the sweetest guy in my life." She laughed at this, then suddenly stopped laughing and turned away for a moment, not wanting Fowler to see what was in her eyes. Then, facing him again, she said, "Okay. Tell me more about sugar."

They were nearing the house. Courage was already waiting for them at the back door. Fowler said, "If there's anything good about sugar, it's that it's easier to find than fat, because the test for sugar is that it's sweet."

"My pop-in-the-toaster-tart," Karen said. "And my donut at work. And of course the sugar coated pops every morning."

"Exactly," Fowler said. "The pop-in-the-toaster-tarts and sugar coated pops and especially all those sugar-filled drinks like sodas and juices.

And so, since The Power of One is geared for real life and based on commonsense, the test for sugar is, if something's sweet and it's not a fruit, then it's sugar. And the strategy says, *As much as possible, depending on the circumstances and the situation, we stay away from sugar.*"

"What about sugar substitutes?" Karen asked.

"Now that you know about creativity, you give me the answer to that question."

Karen first shrugged, then slowly said, "The strategy says stay away from sugar. A substitute is not the same thing, it's not sugar. So if the substitute has no fat, and I've eaten breakfast, then using my creativity, I'd say, thank God for sugar substitutes!"

Fowler nodded. "If you follow the rest of the strategies, and stay, to the degree you're comfortable, within their guidelines, then sugar substitutes are one way to satisfy your sweet tooth."

"There's another?" Karen said.

"There sure is," Fowler answered her, stepping back onto the porch. "And we'll get to it later."

CHAPTER
18

"**B**ut before we look at other ways to satisfy your sweet tooth," Fowler said, opening the door for Karen and allowing Courage to dash in first, "let me take you on another tour of my restaurant."

"I'll just go see if Gabe's up," Karen said.

When she stepped into the kitchen a few minutes later, she had Gabe in her arms. Janice steered herself in as well, with Courage tight at her side.

"Finished?" Fowler said to Janice, taking the empty coffee cup she held in her hand.

"For now," she said. Turning to Karen, she added, "For the past hour I was on-line with five people from four countries in two time zones. All of us are worried about the rush to genetically modified foods. If I had my way there'd be very little of it commercially available, at least until the studies are more conclusive."

Gabe let out a tentative cry. Karen said, "I'd better change him."

"May I help?" Janice asked.

"Of course."

Karen carried Gabe to the spare bedroom and laid him on the bed. While Janice played with his hands, she changed his diaper, noting, "He's relaxed with you. That's unusual for him."

"He's a quiet baby, isn't he?"

"Only with some people," Karen answered, smiling at the expression of delight Janice wore as Gabe reached for her fingers.

When they returned to the kitchen they found Fowler whistling along to a tune on the radio. "I'm ready for that tour of your restaurant," Karen said, placing Gabe, now practicing his bubble-blowing, into his seat. Janice parked her chair next to the baby, then reached for one of her math books from the shelf behind her. She put it on the table, but left it unopened, opting instead to tickle one of Gabe's feet.

Fowler said to Karen, "Good, that tour's just about to leave. And then we'll cook three Power of One breakfasts."

Karen stepped behind the counter.

Fowler opened the cupboard doors. "Okay, this time let's start with what you do see." Then he added, "And I also think it's time to tell you about strategy number four."

"Yes!" Karen said. "Okay, tell you what I do see. Well... Hey! A jar of sugar!"

"That's right. A jar of sugar. Remember what I told you — the strategies are designed to be tailored to each of us, *to fit our individual needs,* because we're not all stamped from the same mold. So even though the strategies give all of us identical guidelines, the way we each apply those guidelines will vary. And in my case, though the strategy says to have as little sugar as possible, I personally enjoy a cup of tea in the afternoon."

"So very British."

"Yes. It is. And I also refuse to have my tea without sugar."

Karen, about to go on with Fowler's tour, suddenly realized that what he'd just said was, to her, almost unbelievable. She turned to him. "You said that so quickly, and gave it so little importance. But just think what it means. You said you *allow* yourself sugar in your tea. That it's *your choice.* That this is the way you tailored this strategy to fit your needs."

"Exactly," Fowler said. "I'm still following the strategy. But I do it on my own terms. I refuse to struggle and so I don't."

Karen shook her head in amazement. "The Power of One isn't a diet, is it? It really doesn't have that *all-or-nothing diet mentality*. It is a guideline. One the entire nation's been missing. It's a return to nutritional sanity."

"I couldn't have put it better myself," Fowler said, smiling.

"So the sugar in your tea is how you manage to accommodate your sweet tooth, right?"

"Nope. That's just sugar in my tea. My sweet tooth get's accommodated in other ways."

"How?"

"Later. What else do you see?"

Karen continued looking in the cupboard. "I see that bottle of olive oil."

"Right. And?"

"And that's it, that's all I see that applies to the first three strategies — as little fat as possible, as little sugar as possible, and eating breakfast every day. Of course there are also all those cans of nonstick spray, whole wheat bread and multigrain rolls, cans of chickpeas and beans and lentils and tuna and salmon and tomatoes, and all different types of pastas and bags of rice."

Turning to the fridge and deli counter she continued, "And there's plenty of fruit and vegetables and salad and one percent milk and all those fat-reduced cheeses and yogurt and raw eggs and hard-boiled eggs. Whew!" Then Fowler motioned her to the freezer. She looked inside and said, "Here's all types of frozen vegetables and packages of turkey breasts and ground turkey and chicken breasts and veal and ground meat and — meals, a thousand premade meals."

"Not exactly a thousand."

"Fifty?"

"Maybe." Then Fowler said, "Okay, now that you saw what is there, I want you to tell me what isn't there."

Karen turned to Janice. "He is strange, isn't he?"

Janice, though, was focused on Gabe, listening to one of his wet-blabbered stories while he held her thumb in his hand. Karen got her attention by saying, "Janice, your father wants to know what I don't see in his restaurant."

"What you don't see," Janice replied, turning to Karen, "what you'll never see here, is any snack or meal made in a factory."

"What?"

"That's right," Fowler said. "Remember I told you there were two kinds of foods. First there's the natural food that's grown and raised and caught by our farmers and ranchers and fishermen—the wonders of the world. And then there's the food that our culture, The Enemy, makes from those natural products.

"And so, what you'll never see in my restaurant, my haven, are factory-cooked foods." He paused, then repeated with even more emphasis, "There are no factory-prepared meals here. No factory-prepared snacks or gravies or any of that stuff. It doesn't matter whether they come in bags or pouches or boxes or jars or cans. It doesn't matter if they're made to be eaten cold or warm or on the run. In this restaurant, everything we have, within reason, *is as close to natural as possible*. I won't have anything here that has ingredients I can't pronounce, items whose source I can't figure out. And that's not to say I don't want anything that comes in cans or boxes or bags or jars. It's not the containers I object to, it's what's in them. In my haven, as much as possible, I want the *primary source of food*, and not the food our culture processes it into."

Karen said, "No factory-made snacks or meals," then winced. "In my kitchen I have them all. The frozen meals. The ones in cans. Pouches of prepared pastas and rice. Chips and cookies and everything else under the sun that's greasy and sugar-filled."

Then she suddenly realized what Fowler was getting at, had been getting at all along. "It really is all the same, isn't it? The processed food in my kitchen is the same as the food I get at the fast-food joints or family restaurants or when I order in. Same junk, different names. They're The Enemy's weapons, advertised to the hilt, and aimed right at my house. Right at my family."

"That's exactly what they are," Fowler said. "But we forget that because if we have to put it into a pot or heat it up in the microwave, it feels different. It feels as though we're making it ourselves.

"Look, I'll buy fresh or canned tomatoes, packages of herbs and spices, onions and frozen carrots and green peppers and minced meat. And I'll buy all kinds of pastas, fresh and dry. But I'll never buy factory-made spaghetti and meat sauce, because they can't make it the way I do. As low in fat as possible and as low in sugar as possible and preservative-free. And the same goes for bread." He smiled at Karen. "Remember when you said bread was yours and Gary's problem?"

Karen nodded.

"Well," Fowler said, "the problem is really only bread made from refined flour. White flour. Flour that has all the nutrients worked out of it. So all the excellent breads and rolls, the whole wheat and multigrains and ethnic breads, are great. The only exception to bread is white bread."

"But the French toast *was* made with white bread."

Fowler grinned. "That's because The Power of One is designed to *work for me*. I don't work for it. And since Janice and I like our French toast made with white bread, that's how we make it. And the same with the dough for my pizzas. There too I use white flour. But for me, *that's it*. None of the other breads or rolls I eat are made from refined flour. That's how I've adapted this strategy to my needs, my tastes and circumstances. Because this strategy, like all the others, has to be tailored to fit me and not the other way around. The Power of One is a passion, I'll admit that. It's an excitement. But the one thing it isn't is a religion."

Janice turned to Karen. "After a speech like that, can you tell what strategy number four is?"

"Boy, can I ever. *Strategy number four - I will not bring any factory-made foods or refined flour products into my home.*" Then she added, "Within reason."

"According to your carefully thought-out needs," Fowler said.

"According to my needs," Karen repeated, knowing that up to now her needs said she had to have her kitchen filled with white sandwich breads and prepared meals and snacks — the-eat-right-out-of-the-bag kind, the heat-up kind, the open-the-can-or-pouch-and-throw-it-into-a-pot-and-hope-for-the-best kind. All necessary for those times when she was rushed or tired or just not in the mood to cook.

Then she thought, Why is that? Why can't I also replace that junk with nutritious meals and snacks of my own, the way Fowler does. Fill up my freezer ahead of time, the way his is filled. Put those into the microwave or oven instead of the factory-made stuff. What's so wrong with me that's so right with him? She shook her head. Gary says it's that I'm lazy. Even stupid. But that's not true. It's just that I didn't have the answer. Until this minute, I didn't realize there was another way.

To Fowler she said, "It is a war, isn't it? I'm fighting Them, our Culture. And I'm fighting me! And I think I can defeat them and change me. Make a meal, make it using the strategies, make more than I need — and put what's not used into the freezer. Just one meal. Then another time, maybe the next weekend, make another meal, something different. A big batch of it! And add that to the first. And the same thing with snacks. Those potatoes you make that taste better than french fries, or your mini pizzas, or any of your other snacks. How long could it take before my freezer also starts to look like yours? Before I could also come home in the evening and sort of go shopping there? In the freezer. Pick and choose from the good stuff."

She smiled. "There is a certain excitement to all this, isn't there? Whether you call it the beginning of a journey or fighting a war, it does get the adrenaline pumping." Then she thought, There's even another benefit to this, and said, "You know, if you think about it, not buying any snacks and meals made in a factory means leaving out whole aisles in the grocery store. It might even save money."

"It will," Fowler said. "But that bonus is completely beside the point. The reason for putting this strategy into The Power of One is that it gives us control over our own nutritional lives. It takes that power *away* from The Enemy and places it back in our own hands. This strategy makes me feel *powerful*."

"I think," Janice said to Fowler, "that this strategy was the one you thought about most. It's the one you kept honing, kept digging deeper into. The one that, long after you'd accepted its basic concept, you still found yourself searching through, always trying to discover your bottom-line comfort level."

"You're right," Fowler agreed. "I do it all so unconsciously now, so naturally. But I remember how everything I bought, everything I brought into the restaurant, I analyzed. I thought it through. Tried to duplicate my way to see if I could make it better. Some of the decisions, of course, were simple. The fat-laden garbage and sugar-filled junk was immediately out. But I also experimented with factory-made low-fat meals. Low-fat sauces. Low-fat snacks. All the other low-fat and lite and sugar-free gimmicks The Enemy is continually pumping into our grocery stores. And I found that, for me, most of them were unacceptable. My standards had become too high, my health and my family's health too valuable. And in the end, my methods are better, just as quick, less expensive, and tastier."

Karen, taking notes again, said, "You first developed the strategy, then looked at it degree by degree, item by item, until you came to the point you're at now, what you call your comfort level."

"That's it," Fowler said. Then, walking to the fridge and opening one of its drawers, he added, "Talking about my comfort level, you haven't looked in here yet."

Karen stepped closer. "What's this?" she asked, lifting out a package of meatless, soya-based pepperoni. "This is certainly factory-made."

"That's what I mean about adjusting to your comfort level," Fowler said. "One of my favorite foods used to be pepperoni pizza dripping with fat. And I didn't want to give it up. So I didn't. I still have it, often. But now *I* make it. And it's incredible how simple it is to make. And I make several at a time and freeze them. But to make them the way I like them, I need this product, this factory-made product, which I think is excellent. So I buy it all the time, along with fat-reduced mozzarella cheese and canned pizza sauce and mushrooms and green peppers. And I challenge any store-bought or delivered pizza to a taste test against mine. But mine, unlike theirs, is downright healthy."

"It's so adjustable," Karen said. "The entire Power of One. So *unlike* a diet, letting you move forward gradually, at a pace *you* can live with. *Not at a pace someone else decides.* I only know four strategies so far, but even with that, I don't know if I can ever really eat the way I did before I learned them. Not without feeling that something's wrong. When it's so easy to get..." She looked at her notes. "When it's so easy to gain health—always that, incrementally and continuously, for the rest of your life." Then she added, "And so easy to lose weight. Especially that."

"Not especially that," Fowler said. "Though I have to admit, when I first started this for myself, that was the goal. But I can see now that that goal was shortsighted. With my focus only on losing weight, I was denying myself something that in both the short and long term is much more important. Something that right now, yesterday and today and tomorrow, is more important to my family. And that's health. Mine and Janice's.

"But that doesn't mean I don't know what you're feeling. A blood test is one thing. Seeing your blood pressure go down, your blood sugar stabilize, your cholesterol drop, your chances of heart disease and cancer lessen — at certain times these seem like small potatoes compared to looking in the mirror and beginning to like what you see. That, for me, when it happened — when I was able to look in the mirror and say, there, that's more like it — was exceptional."

CHAPTER

19

"**A**lright," Fowler said. "It's time to eat, to have our lazy Sunday-morning Power of One fantasy breakfast, on a Monday."

"We just talked about food that's factory made, I know that," Karen said, "but what about certain cereals, the fat-free and sugar-free brands, served with skim or one percent milk? Would that be alright?"

"You tell me."

Karen's brow creased. "Well, if they're low in fat and low in sugar, and they're breakfast, and fit my rushed circumstances, then even though they're factory-made, even though they go against the guidelines of one of the strategies, I'd say yes, they would be alright."

"Not just alright," Fowler said, "but excellent, because The Power of One *is based on real life and commonsense*, and when a product is good, it's good. Karen, you have to take a look at what's out there, assess it for its nutritional value, for your lifestyle, for your immediate circumstances — then make your choice."

"It really is simple, isn't it?" Karen said.

Fowler thought a moment before saying, "The Power of One is simple in theory. That's true. And it's simple when it finally becomes second nature, when the thought of the alternative, of the way it used to be, *is impossible*. But at the beginning — no, I don't believe The Power of One, or for that matter, anything worthwhile, anything requiring courage, is simple. And that's why, once the first step is taken, once that first small success is achieved, and then the next, and the next, once you've given The Power of One the time it needs to build momentum, you can proudly hold your head up high in victory."

"At having beaten The Enemy."

"Yes, at having beaten The Enemy," Fowler said. "Okay. Now go all out. Tell me your dream breakfast. And Janice will tell us hers. And I'll tell you mine. Because *each of our Powers of One are different*, uniquely ours, according to our personal tastes. Then together we'll create courageous, creative, and strategic magic."

Karen said, "My dream breakfast, that's easy. What I feel like eating right now is a western omelet with home-fried potatoes and a ton of bacon."

"Okay, let's see you get out of that one," Janice said to Fowler.

"Well, the spuds are on. And they'll be perfection. And the omelet too, you can count on that also being outstanding. And the bacon? Later I'll tell you how you can have the bacon and still be within the strategies, because *no food is left out of The Power of One.* But for today, since bacon doesn't fit into *my* fat-reduced haven, the one I designed for *me*, the best I can do is find you a perfectly acceptable replacement."

"Knowing I can have everything except the bacon," Karen said, "makes the bacon itself seem insignificant."

"Now that," Fowler said, "looking at food from that perspective, is courage." He turned to Janice.

Janice said, "I'll have a cheese omelet."

"Good. And for me, I know exactly what I want. I've been thinking about it all morning — spaghetti and meat sauce with scrambled eggs and turkey balls."

"What?" Karen said.

Janice said to her, "He's not kidding. He can have his dinner in the morning and his breakfast at night, or just pizza three times a day. I've never been able to understand his cravings or his appetite."

Fowler looked at Karen. "To our bodies, food is just a bunch of nutrients. As long as what you're eating follows the strategies, it doesn't matter what label you think the meal should have — breakfast, lunch, dinner, or snack. So let's get to work. We have VIP customers — and we're going to knock their socks off!"

Then in rapid succession he said, "Why don't you start by refilling our glasses with water and lemon wedges, then put the kettle on for tea, then clean a green pepper and a handful of mushrooms, and grab a couple of spuds from the pantry and let's get them peeled."

"Yes sir!" Karen answered.

Working beside her, Fowler took a carton of eggs and two large packages of regular ground beef from the fridge.

"Even I know that that meat is filled with fat," Karen said.

"Watch and learn," Fowler countered. He opened the packages of beef, dropped them into a large pot, set the pot on the stove with the burner adjusted to medium, and began breaking up the meat with a wooden spoon.

Karen, keeping one eye on Fowler, washed the green pepper and mushrooms and diced them, then began to peel the potatoes.

While the meat was browning, Fowler got to work peeling four large onions. "Some of this is for your omelet," he said, "and the rest is for my meat sauce."

"Now what?" Karen asked, when the potatoes were peeled.

"Dice them, then rinse them and zap them in the microwave until they're soft. And while that's happening you can crack open — let's see, three for you, three for Janice, and five for me — that's eleven eggs. Crack 'em. Use only three yolks, and put them all into a large bowl."

Karen said, "You know, you can buy colored egg whites in cartons."

"I know I can," Fowler said. "And I will, just as soon as those cartons start coming out the rear ends of chickens." Once again he stirred the browning meat. Already there was an inch of liquid fat in the pot.

Then he peeled the onions and diced them in the food processor and, with a quick change of blades, sliced four celery stalks.

"Okay," Karen said, "eleven egg whites and three yolks, ready and waiting."

Fowler nodded. "Now put a drop of one percent milk into them, a hefty splash of tobasco, and beat those suckers. And watch what I'm going to do with this meat."

The ground meat was completely browned and sitting in an inch and a half of liquid fat. Fowler put a colander over the sink and poured the meat into the colander, letting the fat drain while he filled the now empty pot with a couple of inches of water. He put the pot back onto the stove and set the burner on high. "Now I'm going to boil the meat for about two minutes," he said. "Then I'll drain it again and boil it again. And drain it again. Then boil it a third time. And when I'm finished there'll be practically *no fat left*. Only the texture and taste of the meat. And I guarantee, when you taste the finished sauce you'll love it. And, because of the amount I'm making, I've got a good ten spaghetti meals here, or two huge lasagnas, or, if I spice it differently and mix in egg whites as a binder, I can use this meat to stuff a dozen green peppers or fill four shepherd's pies."

Karen stared at Fowler. "That's amazing. You've taken the worst of what's out there — and turned it into the best. Fat-reduced meat sauce, fat-reduced lasagna, fat-reduced meat pies and stuffed peppers. Gary and I love that stuff."

Fowler said, "I simply refuse to believe that any meal I want can't be made to be as low in fat as possible. I refuse to believe that it can't fit into the strategies. And when I start with that mind-set, plus a healthy dose of creativity, a good sense of humor — *and no diet mentality* — I always win."

CHAPTER

20

"**O**kay," Fowler said, grabbing two cans of nonstick spray from a shelf over the sink filled with only that item, and handing one of the cans to Karen, "the non-stick pans are in that cupboard. Treat them with respect because that's how they treat me and my waistline—and remember, when you buy your own, you don't have to buy the most expensive brand. No matter the price, they all last the same amount of time and then need to be replaced."

Karen opened the cupboard he'd pointed out, and Fowler, talking quickly, said, "Let's start with one large pan for your spuds, another smaller one for your omelet, another for my turkey balls, and one more for Janice's omelet and then my scrambled eggs. And since we've already got the kettle on and the meat boiling, we're cooking the way I like to cook—like maniacs!"

Karen laughed.

"He's getting ready to blow," Janice said. "I've seen this before. It could be dangerous."

"That's me," Fowler said. "Dangerous!" He twirled his can of nonstick spray into the air, caught it upright in his other hand, snapped off the cover with his thumb, then began to liberally spray first one frying pan, then another, then another.

Janice said, "Go get 'em, killer!"

"Okay," Fowler said to Karen, "let's get those spuds going, and the green pepper and mushrooms and onions. And while you're doing that I'll get the turkey smoking."

Working with a full smile and at an exaggerated pace, Fowler pulled two packages of ground turkey breast from the fridge, ripped open the packages and placed the meat into a bowl. Breaking up the meat with a fork, he said, "I just got another brainstorm. Listen to this." He turned to Janice, winked, then said to Karen, "We talked about creativity, right?"

"Right."

"Well, inside The Power of One there's really two kinds of creativity. The most important kind, the one we already talked about, says, *within your comfort zone,* you'll do whatever has to be done to follow the nutritional road map of the eight strategies."

But before Fowler could continue, Karen asked, "Why do you always begin any discussion of the strategies with the phrase *within your comfort zone?*"

Janice said, "He does that because that was the way he originally devised the strategies, by first constructing the logic of the strategy, understanding the need for it, then applying more and more effort into it while judging how it could become a *part of his life, without interfering with his life.* He used to call it his balancing act."

"That's right," Fowler said. "My balancing act. I also keep talking about the comfort zone because *if any part of the strategies becomes irritating, then it becomes useless, just like a diet.*"

Karen nodded. "So that's why we each create our *own* Power of One. Because we do it the way you did it, first by understanding the reason for the strategy, then by *personalizing it to our individual needs and urges*, like you did with the sugar in your tea."

"Exactly," Fowler replied. "My Power of One is not quite the same as Janice's. And yours will be different from either of ours."

"And with it personalized," Karen said, "it then fits into each of our lives without it being a struggle, the way diets are a struggle — because they leave no room to maneuvre."

"That's right," Fowler said. "And after a while you won't notice it. The Power of One becomes ingrained. Second nature. *It disappears.*"

"It does disappear, doesn't it?" Karen said slowly. "You don't even realize you're working with it anymore. It just becomes the way things are."

Fowler grinned. "For us, it disappeared a long time ago."

"Along with your excess weight," Karen said. She shook her head, then added, "You were saying there are two kinds of creativity. What's the other?"

"The other," Fowler answered, "is this." He opened the cupboard where he kept his herbs and spices and with a flourish and a quick mood change back to overdrive, picked out the garlic powder, pepper, salt, dried dill, sage, and tobasco and Worcestershire sauces and, while tossing into the ground turkey single shakes of one and double shakes of another, said, "*Have fun! Experiment! Don't be afraid!* The only people who can't dance are the ones who won't get onto the dance floor!"

Then he suddenly stopped everything he was doing and, hooding his brows, asked Karen, "Are you sure you're crazy enough to be working in my kitchen?"

Karen, with a quick, sly expression of her own, answered, "I don't know. Why don't you test me!"

Janice said to Gabe, "Watch your mommy. After today she may never be the same."

Fowler, his hands now wrist-deep in the turkey mix, said, "Okay. I don't want you to think. Just follow my instructions, one after the other, without taking a breath. And it's gonna be fast. Ready?"

"Ready!"

"Good." He raised one eyebrow, paused a full five seconds, then, like a drill sergeant barking orders, shouted, "Toss the spuds! Pour part of the egg mixture into the green pepper and mushrooms! Pour half the rest into a bowl! Toss the spuds! Take the kettle off the burner! Toss the spuds! Throw the onions and celery into that pot! Mow the lawn! Toss the spuds!"

Karen kept up with Fowler's instructions until he told her to mow the lawn. Then she threw her hands into the air, laughed at the all-out silliness she and Fowler and Janice were capable of, looked at Janice, looked at Fowler, then, with her face flushed red, laughed again, this time exploding into an out-of-control howl so loud and full that Courage jumped to his feet and with his hackles raised began to bark.

Karen said to Fowler, "I'll mow the lawn and you pave the street and Janice and Gabe will discover new planets and Courage'll—"

The doorbell rang. A moment later someone began to pound on it, and then a deep, loud, furious voice, yelled, "Karen! I know you're in there and I want you to get the hell out! Now!"

CHAPTER
21

Karen pushed her cart up the aisle of the grocery store. Inside the cart were econo-size packages of chips and chocolate cakes, colas and frozen meals and ice cream. To this, she added two boxes of sugar coated pops and two of pop-in-the-toaster-tarts. It was mid-afternoon. The store was crowded. Gabe, buckled into the cart's bright blue baby seat, had his fist around the plastic turnip Fowler had bought him. The last time Karen had seen Fowler was eight days ago, the day Gary had appeared at his door and demanded that she come home.

She reached for another sugarcoated cereal, feeling the heavy sway of fat beneath her arm stretch. Suddenly her eyes met Fowler's. She held his stare for only an instant before quickly steering her cart away from his and around the corner.

At the end of this aisle she looked back to see if he had followed her, but he hadn't. She pressed her jaws together, knowing this wasn't supposed to happen. A moment later she turned her cart back into the aisle to find him. When she saw him moving toward her, she waited.

"Hello," Fowler said.

"Don't you do this at night?" Karen said. "I told myself I didn't have to worry about running into you."

"I changed my schedule."

"Just now? This week? After so many years?"

Fowler shrugged his shoulders. "How are you?"

"I'm fine. Getting back to normal. The situation is working itself out. This last week has been quiet."

"We were worried about you."

"I know. I knew you would be. I'm sorry." In a muted tone she added, "Gary asked me not to see you again. Not to get in touch." All she could be, she knew, was honest. When she'd left Fowler's house she'd gone in the only direction she saw ahead of her, back to the security of hopelessness. She struggled to keep that emotion out of her voice.

Fowler touched her arm. "Why does he keep saying that?"

Karen sighed. "He doesn't like it when I'm with other people, he's always been that way—protective. And now, with the baby..."

"He has a strange way of being protective," Fowler replied.

Karen moved her cart to the side and said quietly, "Fowler, sometimes things happen in a marriage that look one way on the outside and another on the inside. Gary is suspicious by nature, I knew that when I married him. Suspicious and jealous and very private. So he became upset when I met you. You know that. He understood how it happened, though. He just wasn't happy about it. And then when I told him about the things you were teaching me—you know, about nutrition, about The Power of One—it bothered him even more."

"How could learning about nutrition bother him?"

Karen smiled sheepishly. "You're not a doctor, Fowler. But Gary says you think you are. He says you're acting like some mystical know-it-all and thinks there's more to what you're doing than just being helpful. He's worried you're trying to take over my mind, turn me into some sort of follower, like they do in cults. He thinks you might be dangerous."

She knew Fowler could tell she didn't believe a word Gary had said. She went on, though, "He also said that if there was anything wrong with any of the food in this store, they wouldn't be able to sell it."

"Well," Fowler answered her, "at least there, on a certain level, he's right."

"He is?"

"Of course. There's no food in this store that could be labeled poison. No warning on anything that says, eat too much of this and you'll eventually get blocked arteries or diabetes or cancer and die." He paused, then asked, "What about your weight? Did you tell him The Power of One would help with that?"

Karen nodded.

"And?"

"When it comes to my weight, Gary only believes one thing — that I'm fat because I'm lazy and stupid. He said from now on I should stand while I eat so the food won't get stuck in my stomach. So it'll go through without attaching itself to me."

Fowler's expression remained blank. "Where did he learn that bit of wisdom?"

"I don't know. He also said I should get an ab machine, the kind they advertise on tv. And that I should do that for an hour or two a day."

"An hour or two?"

Karen smiled wryly. "He made me do sit-ups last night. He was holding my feet and yelling at me, but I couldn't do even one. I couldn't lift myself off the ground."

"What did he say about that?"

"The usual."

Fowler reached out to Gabe, saying, "Hey, little guy. How're you doing?" But Gabe was more interested in the wall of brightly colored boxes than in Fowler. Fowler said to Karen, "What about Gary's weight, how's that?"

"He's big," Karen answered, "like me. Maybe sixty pounds overweight. But it's different on a man. Gary says women like their men big, that it gives them a sense of security, and that he sees women staring at him all the time." Once more she shrugged her shoulders, then added, "Fowler, I know he's not perfect, but I need Gary, for a lot of reasons. So does Gabe. We'd both be in trouble without him. And in his own way, he loves me. I know that."

"I'm glad he does," Fowler replied, glancing at the items in Karen's cart.

Karen, watching him, said, "That's why I didn't want you to see me. I didn't want you to know what I was buying."

"Why not? Gary says all this is fine, otherwise they wouldn't be allowed to sell it. And that all you have to do to get slim, and healthy too, I suppose, is eat standing up."

In a very soft voice, Karen said, "I know he's wrong. And I know you're right. And I know everything about The Power of One is right. But, Fowler, there are all kinds of people in this world, and some people, like me... we're the kind who just can't..." She paused.

"Can't what?" Fowler pressed. "Can't make The Power of One work?"

"That's right. I'm one of those people it won't work for. I know that from my own history. Any kind of success with losing weight passes me by, rushes by as though I were a big fat rock in a stream. And I've learned to accept that. Maybe Gary knows what he's talking about. Maybe when it comes to losing weight, I am stupid."

Fowler reached into Karen's cart and lifted out a tub of chocolate ice cream and said, "Tell me about this. What's in it?"

"Fat," Karen answered quickly, having thought about it long before Fowler asked the question.

"And?"

"And sugar, lots of it. And the fat and sugar make it taste good." She'd thought about that too. Used that obvious truth to get it from the grocery store freezer into her cart.

"That's right," Fowler said. "It does taste good. And I also love ice cream, and I eat it regularly. But even though it tastes good, how did you feel when you put it into your cart?"

"Lousy," Karen admitted, shaking her head. "Weak and angry and stupid."

"Why did you feel that way?"

"Because I know it's garbage. And this is garbage too," she added, pointing to the cereals. "And the drinks and the frozen meals. None of it fits into the strategies."

"Then it's working," Fowler said.

"What?"

"It's working. The Power of One is working. The knowledge of the battle is in you now, and that knowledge has gotten to you. The fact of the war has gotten to you. It's gone from your brain to your emotions. You can feel the fight. *Feel your loss of control.* And there's nothing you can do to stop that. You can still buy this kind of food. And eat it. But you can never be the same with it. In fact, you can never really enjoy it again, not until you know all the strategies, not until you can slot even *this* food comfortably into the strategy it belongs — eat it, the way I do, knowing all you have to know. And then you'll savor it. I guarantee it. But not until then."

Fowler smiled. "Just the knowledge of it, just the fact of the war, and the outline of The Power of One, has already changed your life."

Karen, her voice barely a whisper, said, "It has changed my life. There were times during this past week when I wasn't sure whether it was knowing what they, the manufacturers of this junk, are doing to me, that got me so mad, or if it was you. The fact that you opened my eyes to it, that was upsetting me. But what I know for sure is that I can't stop reciting the first four strategies as though they were a mantra. I see them in my mind like your neon sign. As little fat as possible. As little sugar as possible. Eat breakfast. Stay away from factory-cooked meals and snacks, and do all of it within my comfort zone. Without feeling any of my *diet guilts or frustrations*.

"Because of you I know it's me against them. The Enemy. I know that. And I know that The Enemy is getting rich at the same time that he's slowly but surely killing me. Now when I drive down the street and see the fast-food places or hear food ads on the radio or see them on tv, I think, You're out to get me! You've turned making me fat into advertising science. Moneymaking science. *You're destroying my health and my family's health for the sake of a buck.*

"And it was you who did this to me, Fowler. You and Janice opened my eyes. A couple of weeks ago I would have bought this ice cream and felt as though I was buying comfort. Even excitement. Taking home a friend. Now I bought it and I know I'm letting The Enemy into my house. And I feel like a traitor."

"Traitor?" Fowler said, his eyes widening. "That's perfect! That's the perfect word, the perfect description." Then he added, "Traitor to who, though?"

"To me?" Karen said hesitantly.

Fowler looked Karen in the eyes. "Do you have time for a coffee?"

CHAPTER

22

Fowler and Karen went to a coffee bar tucked into one corner of the store and ordered two coffees and two glasses of water with lemon wedges. Gabe was sitting quietly in the baby seat. Karen parked the shopping cart next to the table and took a biscuit from her bag and gave it to him, then turned her attention to Fowler.

Fowler said, "I'd like to tell you something that has nothing to do with The Enemy or the war or The Power of One, but everything to do with my life and the way I live it."

Karen nodded.

"There was a time when my life was a lot like yours," Fowler began. "When I did whatever I needed to do—just to get through the day. I ate too much and drank too much and thought of food and alcohol as my friends, my love-hate, hold-me-upright and keep-me-going friends. And I thought of the reflection in my mirror as the enemy. I disgusted myself— blamed myself for my failed marriage, Janice's medical condition. Everything. And the wheels kept going around. There was no end and no way out."

"Lately I feel as though I'm floating in space," Karen said. "That I can't grab hold of anything solid. That I'm moving further and further away and I can't stop it, don't know how to get back to solid ground."

"I know it well," Fowler replied. "It all seems so hopeless and complicated. You don't know where to start to change it or how to start or when to start. You don't know even in theory what the first step is."

"That's exactly it," Karen whispered, leaning forward and listening to Fowler's every word. Suddenly she sat upright and said, "You're not going to tell me The Power of One will change all that, are you? That losing weight is the answer to all my problems?"

"No," Fowler said. "The Power of One can work magic, it can go beyond what it initially presents itself to be. But it won't work in a vacuum. It won't work if you just sort of discover it while you're floating out there in space and pick it out of the air and hang on to it, without having a foundation to tie it to, to cement it and you into place."

Once again Karen leaned forward.

Fowler said, "What happened for me was that over time, all of my grasping, hoping, needing—all of my emotions—began to form into a new feeling, a new understanding, a new way of looking at my life. At first this understanding was unclear, coming to me in little snatches — like single words outside a sentence. Then it began to take shape and I realized that what I needed in my crazy life was just one thing —simplicity."

"Simplicity?"

"Yes. Just that. What I needed was to bring my life into focus. Drain the swamp it had become. And I'm going to tell you what I did to do that, so maybe you can do something similar. Create a similar, simple, solid structure for your life."

Karen nodded, urging him to continue.

"What I did," Fowler said, "was reduce every element of my life into just three priorities. First my family, which is Janice, her emotional and physical health. Then me, my emotional and physical health. Then my work. And that's it. Those three priorities cover every aspect of my life, every part that I had before I gained control of it, every part now, while I'm in control, and every part I'll ever have in the future. Those three priorities cover everything. And put all the elements of my life into their proper order.

"Now, each day I know I have three things to take care of. I can list them in a second and focus on them throughout the day and hang my hat on them at night. The structure is simple. And comforting. First my family, then me, then my work."

For a moment Karen was silent, then she said, "For me it would be first Gabe."

"And Gary."

"My family?"

"Right. Your family. Their physical and emotional well-being, which could be spiritual as well as psychological. You take care of it now, I know you do, but you just don't have it prioritized. So you're fighting the fires when they break out, instead of working on fire prevention."

"You mean between Gary and me?"

"That would fit in there, in priority number one."

My first priority, then," Karen said, "the first thing I would think of when I woke up in the morning, would be my family, Gabe and Gary, their emotional and physical well-being."

"Right."

"And the second priority?"

"The second priority," Fowler said, "is you. Your emotional and physical well-being. That's how I do it. How I see it. My family, Janice, is first, because she takes up most of the space in my heart. But there's room left over in my heart for me. I've learned to give me what I need for my physical and emotional well-being too. I've learned how to become my own friend. After Janice, my priority is now me, and in fact the two priorities go together because— "

"Because if you forgot about you," Karen said, "there would be no you to give to Janice."

"Exactly. My priority of me is really part of my priority for her. And I don't mean just my physical health, but also my emotional health. Without that, I'd be less effective for her. So in all the ways I tell her I love her, I also tell myself, in other ways, that I've got me as a friend now too."

"And then there's your work."

"Right. I need it. We all do, I guess, to pay the bills. And I like it, I... thrive on it. And I put a lot of effort into it. But it's priority number three — of three. It used to be number one. Then number two, after Janice. Then I got smart and put it where it belongs — last. Think about what I'm saying, though. My work is not unimportant. To me it's very important. But it's still the last priority of three, which, in so many ways, all tie together.

"So now, with this order of priorities straight in my head, listed in front of me before I've even gotten out of bed, the day ahead becomes clear. The wheels are still spinning, but they're spinning the way I want them to. And now at the end of the day I can look back and ask, Did I do what I wanted for Janice? Did I contribute to her emotional and physical well-being? And then I can ask the same for me, did I do what I needed to do during the day to contribute to my emotional and physical well-being? And last, before I doze off, I can review what I did for my work. And ask myself if I did anything there I can be proud of."

Karen said, "For me, then, I would start by thinking about Gary and Gabe."

"Yes. And it works the same way for Gary. His number-one priority would be you and Gabe. He would begin his day thinking about you, your emotional and physical well-being, in the same way you would be thinking about his."

"We'd both get what we needed from each other."

"Exactly. But even that has to begin somewhere."

"With me, you mean?"

"That's right. Start it for yourself. Begin the process. You don't need anyone's permission or anyone's involvement. The process begins with adjusting the thoughts in your head."

"Prioritize," Karen said. "My family. Me. My work. Then if Gary wants, if I can talk to him, explain it to him the way you just explained it to me, he would do the same."

"That's the way it would work," Fowler said. "You'd focus on him and he'd focus on you. And your second priority in this world, the one after your family, the one that's so important because it makes it possible to keep your family as your number-one priority, is you. And in that priority is your emotional health and your physical health."

"And that's where you brought in The Power of One," Karen said. "It fits into your second priority."

"And my first, for Janice's health."

Karen leaned back into her seat. After a moment's pause, she said, "I feel as though I'm in the middle of a puzzle that's quickly being solved."

CHAPTER

23

Though she spoke to them twice on the telephone, the first chance Karen had to see Fowler and Janice again was six days after meeting Fowler in the grocery store. This time she drove to their house and on the way over thought, For once at least, they're in for a pleasant surprise.

Janice opened the front door.

Karen smiled.

Janice stared.

Fowler, wearing gardening gloves and carrying a spade, came up behind Karen, saying, "I saw you drive up." When she turned to face him he reacted with a single word. "Wow."

She was dressed in a printed skirt and white blouse and blue jacket. Her hair, newly trimmed and tinted, was now shorter, tighter to her face and more appealing. She had put on makeup and her nails were polished. But most of all there was a new air about her.

"You're glowing," Janice said approvingly. "As though you're being lit from within."

"Thank you," Karen replied. "I feel that way—lit from within."

"I'd say it looks more like you won a lottery," Fowler said.

"To a certain extent I have," Karen answered. "But this lottery has nothing to do with money and everything to do with life."

"Come on in," Janice said.

Fowler, leaving his spade and gloves and boots by the front door, reached for Gabe.

In the kitchen Karen pulled out a chair and sat, while Fowler placed Gabe into his seat. Then he went behind the counter and returned with three glasses of water with lemon wedges.

Janice, touching Gabe's hand, shaking it lightly, said to Karen, "What did you mean when you said you won a lottery that has nothing to do with money and everything to do with life?"

"Well," Karen answered, "you probably know that I met Fowler."

Janice nodded.

"And that he told me about the way he'd prioritized his life."

Janice turned to her father. "You didn't tell me that."

Fowler shrugged and turned to Karen. "All I told Janice was that we went through the store a second time and picked out replacements for the food you chose. I thought I'd leave anything else for you to say, if you wanted."

"Thank you," Karen whispered. Then she explained to Janice what Fowler had told her. To Fowler she said, "In just a few weeks, between The Power of One and your list of Life Priorities, you've given me more to think about than I've had to think through in my entire thirty-two years. Now, finally, I'm beginning to understand what it means to have my priorities straight."

"If I helped, then I'm pleased," Fowler said.

"You helped alright. And you're still helping." Karen reached into her purse and took out her journal. "My first decision was that I'm going to take control of my life—move it, without telling Gary, from his hands to mine. And at the same time work on our marriage.

"It's a big order, I know. But I think I can do it. I think I can focus on both my family and myself, together. And part of focusing on myself is choosing my own friends and deciding what's important to me. And I want the two of you as friends, even if, for a while at least, it's better for me not to tell that to Gary."

"Those aren't just some small adjustments to your life, they're major changes," Janice said. "Don't you think that sooner or later Gary's going to find out?"

"Yes. He will. In fact, I'm planning on telling him myself about the priorities and The Power of One. Just not quite yet. You see, with my first priority of caring for him, for my family, as my focus, I'll only tell him at a time when the discussion won't turn into an argument. I want my telling him to be positive, for both of us. And I'm laying the groundwork for that now, not just hoping it'll happen.

"In the last five days or so, since figuring out how these new priorities could work for me, I've become exceptionally good to Gary. Caring and loving. And frankly, at the moment, I don't think he knows what to make of it. He's been quiet. I think he's trying to understand."

Fowler said, "It's hard to challenge a change that obviously makes life better. No one can easily start an argument over, 'Why are you being so good to me?'"

"That's exactly it," Karen said. "It is better now. More peaceful. I keep saying to myself—remember your priorities. And the next thing I say is, Okay, what can I do today, now, this minute, to make Gary's emotional and physical state better? And then I do it, something, anything, even if it's just a kiss on the cheek." She laughed lightly. "The poor guy is perplexed by all of it, by my new attitude toward him and my attitude toward myself. And all he's seen so far is what shows on the surface. When it comes to me, right now, most of the changes are happening beneath my skin."

"Go on," Fowler said. "You can't make a statement like that and stop there."

Karen said, "I've decided to make The Power of One a permanent part of my life and Gary's, whether he knows it or not." She held up her journal. "I want to understand each of the strategies, then begin applying them to my life the same way you did when you first developed them, *by working with each one slowly, letting it adapt to me while I adapt to it.* Letting my comfort level be maintained while my excitement grows, with no *diet anxieties*, none of the *diet mentality* that I hate."

She paused. Then, with her words tumbling through a laugh, she said, "I've started it already, with just the first four strategies, and in five days I've lost two and a half pounds! This is the first time I've ever lost weight without being on a diet, by *eating* my weight off, and I feel unbelievably wonderful! Even my friend, Sue, from work, noticed the change. Yesterday she stopped by my desk and said I looked great and there was something different about me. She saw me eating a meal I brought from home, something I've never done before, so I told her about The Power of One, all that I know so far, especially that it's not a diet—and she wants to try it too." Karen paused to catch her breath. "Of course Gary doesn't know what I'm doing. But when it comes to the food in our house, that's all left up to me, anyway."

She shook the journal in Fowler's direction. "Now I need to know what I'm missing. I want to learn the last four strategies." But before Fowler could say anything, she added, her tone dropping, "First, though, I have a confession to make. This past week, another thing I realized was that when I first told you I wanted to learn about The Power of One, that I'd found the necessary courage to do that, I was wrong."

"How could you have been wrong?" Janice asked. "That's exactly what you said—'I want to learn The Power of One'. How could you say that and *not* have the courage to do it?"

Karen shook her head. "Because that's what we do. That's what overweight people do. We lie to ourselves about courage."

Fowler nodded.

Karen caught Fowler's expression and said to him, "You knew what was happening, didn't you? You knew I was lying to myself about making an honest attempt at controlling my weight."

"I am you," Fowler replied.

"I don't understand," Janice said. "How could you have been lying to yourself?"

Karen sighed. "The lie. *It's how we protect ourselves*, what we project to the world. It's the mask between what we *wish* we could do and what we *believe* we can do. We say we will lose the weight, but in our hearts know we won't. So we don't even try. We just lie about it, lie about the effort to ourselves and to others, sometimes knowingly and sometimes unknowingly. And then fail."

Fowler, looking at Janice, said, "What we do is attempt to try, but don't attempt to succeed, and so we don't. We *sabotage* our efforts, *pretend the sabotage is not there*, then fail, saying, 'I tried, but for me, for some reason, it just didn't work'. Then we walk away until the next time."

"That's it exactly," Karen whispered.

For a long moment there was silence.

Karen lifted her glass of water to her lips and took several slow swallows, then put the glass back on the table.

"I don't know if there's anything more simple to describe, and more complicated to accomplish, than losing weight," Fowler said. "It's true that for some people, being overweight might be a medical problem and they need medical help. And for others it could be a psychological problem, a childhood trauma that's at the root of it, and they need help to recover from that.

"But for most of us, most of the nation, the problem of being overweight comes from only one source." In a booming, announcer-style voice he said, "Attention! Attention every overweight person on the planet. Eat less calories than your body needs — and you'll lose weight!" Then he solemnly dipped his head and said, "Thank you."

Karen said, "The Power of One will do it."

"Yes. It will," Fowler agreed. "But it's not a magic pill. You can't try to lift that glass of water. You can only lift it."

Karen looked at Fowler, then at the glass of water in front of her. She put her fingers around it and, after a long, reflective pause, lifted it. And with the glass aloft, she slowly said, "You're right. I can't *try* to *lift* the glass. I can only lift it. And I can't try The Power of One. *I can only live it.*"

"That's the only way," Fowler said. "You can't try it. It's not a change of clothing. It's not something that can be tried on, checked for its fit, then tossed and forgotten. Once the knowledge is in you, once you understand *why* you're overweight, *who* the Enemy is, and *how* each of the strategies works, you can only, to the degree that you need or want or adjust to for the circumstance, live it, or knowingly, *with your knowledge and consent, ignore it.* But you can't try it for a while or fail at it over time. It's not a piece of clothing or an exam, not something that has an end."

"Live it. Or knowingly ignore it," Karen repeated.

Fowler nodded. "Okay, enough of this seriousness." He lifted his glass of water, took a good swallow, and, tilting the glass in Karen's direction, said, "Are you ready to learn the next strategy?"

CHAPTER

24

Fowler turned to Janice, saying, "*And strategy number five is?*"

"*Water.*"

"Water?" Karen said.

"That's it," Fowler answered. "A one-word strategy that means so much I don't know where to begin."

"Believe it or not," Janice said, "this is the strategy that took him the longest to figure out."

"But I've heard about this one before," Karen said, putting Gabe's pacifier back into his mouth. "We're supposed to drink water. A certain amount of water."

"Eight glasses," Janice said.

"That's right," Karen answered. "Eight glasses of water."

Fowler was shaking his head. "If you have to put a number on it, then eight is as good as any. That's the number that's always bandied about and that's the number I also work around. But remember, I'm not counting anything—not calories or grams or pounds or glasses of water or anything. Nothing about The Power of One is set in stone. If one day I drink six eight-ounce glasses of water and the next day eleven, then that's what it is. This strategy, like all the rest, has to fit into my life, and not the other way around." He smiled as though he was holding back on a secret, then lifted his glass into the air. "Let me tell you about water. The little I know."

In a mock whisper, Janice said to Karen, "He knows it all. Probably more than the so-called experts."

"I know," Karen said back. "I've thought about that. It's because he's living it, walking the walk."

"Water," Fowler said, "is our body's most important nutrient, for a whole slew of scientific reasons, none of which I'm going to go into. Instead, what I'm going to do is go back to my old clunker. And if in that car, carbohydrates are the fuel, then water is its internal carwash. A cleaning agent with a miraculous kick, one that's able to not only flush out everything that needs to be flushed, but also power the reaction, the way oxygen powers fire. Water takes care of our insides and outsides, our internal organs and our skin. Water, plain old water, is one of the keys to turning that clunker into a hot new Ferrari."

"Just water?" Karen said.

"Just water. Plain old water — with a twist of lemon or splash of lime. But water. Nothing carbonated and nothing with sugar or caffeine."

"So all I have to do is drink water?" Karen asked.

Fowler nodded. "That's all you have to do. But don't be fooled by how simple it seems, because it's not."

Janice said, "That's what happened to him at the beginning. He just said, 'I have to drink water' — then forgot about it and went on with the other strategies."

"It's because it seems so easy," Fowler said. "I just accepted it, then basically ignored it, sort of shrugged it into my life without digging deeper into it. I didn't bother focusing on it the way I did with the other strategies."

"Tell her what happened," Janice said.

"I'd gotten all the other strategies down pat. After years of hit-and-miss, of experimenting, of highs and lows and then of going wild with creativity, I'd reached the point where I was comfortable with *my* degree of focus and participation with all the other strategies. I didn't have to think about them anymore. I was living The Power of One to the point where it had grown invisible."

Karen said, "That's another key. After making the right choices and after being prepared, *it's a matter of sticking with it until it becomes second nature.* Until it becomes a positive new habit, one that replaces all the old negative ways. It's got to become so ingrained that it disappears, the way it has for you, and then becomes a part of your life—for the rest of your life."

"That's right," Fowler said. "And by that time, that's what had happened to me — except for this strategy of drinking water, I was *living* The Power of One. And at that point the effect of seeing my results, and letting the excited feeling that came from those results push me into working for even greater results, had been pounding away at me so much that I'd already regained my health and lost most of my extra weight. For me, at that point, my weight was where I figured it would stay. And I was more than just pleased with it — I was thrilled.

"But I'd never focused on the water. I just drank it when I was thirsty — and ignored it the rest of the time. Then I began to think about it and I wondered, Just how much water is eight glasses? And what does it mean to actually drink that much? So I filled an eight-glass pitcher of water and in just one day realized, Hey, this is a lot of water and I'm having trouble getting it all down. So I focused."

"He became creative," Janice said.

"That's right. I knew I liked the taste of lemon, so I began with that. I put lemon wedges into my glass. And that was better. For me, much better. Then, to make things even simpler, I began using lemon juice from a jar, splashing it into a pitcher filled with water, and keeping the pitcher close at hand. But I still wasn't drinking eight glasses. Not easily. Not at a level that I found comfortable."

"He still had to think about it," Janice said. "And he likes to have everything about The Power of One flow, be a part of his world without any thought, so he can ignore it and get on with the rest of his life."

"That's right. And it was bothering me — because it seems so simple. So I focused harder and I thought, How would it be if I replaced my orange juice in the morning with water— with my pitcher filled with cold, lemon-flavored water. So I tried it and found that, for me, the taste of the lemon, first thing in the morning, completely changed the water into a drink that I found not just tasty, but also cleansing. It had the effect of cleaning my palette, as if preparing it for the new day. And I liked that.

"And when I started drinking my lemon-flavored water first thing in the morning, I had no trouble drinking eight glasses. In fact, I found myself often refilling my eight-glass pitcher by noon. And by also keeping a bottle of water in my car and carrying around another with me in the garden, by the end of the day I might have had twelve or thirteen or more glasses. All without trouble. Without a thought. All within my comfort level. But remember, except for that time while I was focusing on the strategy, experimenting with it, deciding how to best tailor it to fit my needs and my life, I don't count glasses."

"Tell her the rest," Janice said impatiently.

Fowler said, "What I also discovered— "

"He was amazed," Janice said.

"Yes, I was truly amazed. Because after figuring out how to apply this strategy to my life, I found that those last few extra pounds I was carrying, pounds I was fully and happily prepared to live with, started to come off."

"Come off?" Karen said.

"Yes! Within weeks of drinking my lemon-flavored, eye-opening, palette-cleansing, first-thing-in-the-morning, then-for-the-rest-of-the-day-sipping water, the extra pounds began to melt away, pound after pound, week after week, until they were gone. Just gone.

"Don't get me wrong. Water by itself won't cause weight-loss. *But it's a necessary addition to all the other strategies, giving them the extra boost they need.*" Fowler grinned. "Until I tried it, I never even suspected there was anything else I could do with The Power of One that would impress me. But there was. And it was the addition of water."

He lifted his glass to Karen. "To this simplest, most logical of strategies — good old water. It's truly astounding. Now let's eat."

CHAPTER

25

Fowler casually leaned back in his chair, crossed his arms over his chest, looked Karen in the eyes, and after a moment's pause, said to her, "But before we eat, I have an important question to ask you."

"Okay."

"Are you hungry?"

"Am I hungry? Me? Of course I'm hungry! I'm always hungry. I'm always starving!"

"Good," Fowler replied. "That's good. What's not so good is that today is one of my lazy days. In fact, right now I'm so lazy I don't even want to get out of my chair. But I still want a great meal, one that follows all the strategies, and I want it in five minutes."

Janice smiled.

Karen said to her, "It sounds as though he's setting me up for something."

"I am," Fowler replied. "You're still my sous-chef, right?"

"Yes sir, mister sir," Karen answered, saluting.

"Good. Then I want you to go to the bank and await further instructions."

Janice laughed. "He means his energy bank. The freezer."

Karen stood and stepped behind the counter and opened the freezer door.

Fowler said, "You can see that everything is either labeled or wrapped in cellophane, so you can tell what it is. So what I want is a smorgasbord of tastes. A bit of everything."

"A tasting tray," Karen said.

"Exactly. A tasting tray for three. And remember, I'm hungry, and so is Janice, and you're starving. Right? Wasn't that the word you used?"

"You'd better believe it," Karen said, reaching into the freezer. She took out the first of the packages. "We'll start with a couple of slices of veal loaf and some turkey balls."

"Find the filet of halibut," Janice said. "It's cleaned and spiced and ready to be steamed, and will only take a couple of minutes. And it's delicious."

"Go for my vegetable rice too," Fowler added. "We'll need a couple of containers of that."

"Halibut, vegetable rice, fried potatoes," Karen said, as she took the packages from the freezer.

Janice said, "Don't forget the eggplant parmesan. And the lasagna."

"And a container of meat sauce," Fowler said.

"I also need a stuffed pepper," Janice said. "I just have to have a stuffed green pepper."

Karen began to laugh.

"And don't forget the vegetables," Fowler said. "I want to see a yellow one and an orange one and at least two shades of green."

"Okay, okay!" Karen said. "There's enough here for an army. You can stop your hollering."

Moving about the kitchen as though she'd been raised in it, Karen found a large microwaveable container and, unwrapping everything, put the eggplant parmesan, vegetable rice, potatoes, turkey balls, veal loaves, stuffed green peppers, and lasagna into it. She covered the container and, along with the container of meat sauce, put it into the microwave, set the timer, and pressed start. Then she took out a large pot and steamer, poured in a triple serving of the frozen mixed vegetables, got that going, and, in a smaller pot, did the same for the halibut. Then she said, as though talking to herself, "That meat sauce has to go on something." And she put up another pot of water for pasta.

Janice said, "You know, I wasn't even hungry. But just hearing that list of food has gotten my juices flowing."

"I can hardly believe it," Karen said. "One incredible meal, coming up in five minutes. Even if we ordered in, it would take longer than that." Then she said, "*It's preparation. That's the key. Take advantage of your energy when you have it. Use it. And save it.*"

Fowler said, "Now all we need is more water."

"Oops. The water." Karen refilled the glasses, then said, "What's next, boss?"

"Next," Fowler replied, "I want you to tell me you're still starving."

Karen laughed. "Of course I'm still starving! I'm always starving. Starving is a part of me, like an extra leg, like the horns on a big fat moose! It goes where I go, does what I do. Leads the way and leads my life!"

"We already told you, though, that a healthy appetite is a sign of good health."

"Then I am one unbelievably healthy—and fat—"

"I'm also hungry," Janice said, cutting in.

"Hungry? Or starving?" Karen wanted to know.

"Just hungry."

"What about you?" Karen said to Fowler. "Are you hungry or starving?"

Fowler said, "I also have a healthy appetite. And I'm also hungry. In fact, at this moment I'm very hungry. But starving? No. And we'll talk about that, about your starving. But not now. Now I want to eat. And," he said, as the microwave began to beep, "suddenly I've got a ton of energy, so I'll serve the meal." He stood and motioned for Karen to take her seat, then went behind the counter.

Karen watched as he first put a good amount of pasta into the boiling water, then took down a serving platter and two plates from the cupboard, and lined the three dishes side by side. Next he took the steaming hot food from the microwave and into the serving platter placed a healthy section of eggplant parmesan, a good cupful of vegetable rice, part of the fried potatoes, five turkey balls, a slice of veal loaf, a serving of lasagna, one stuffed green pepper, a hefty amount of the now ready pasta crowned with the meat sauce, and a heaping quantity of the mixed vegetables.

Then into one of the plates he put the filet of halibut, a cupful of vegetable rice, and a cup of mixed vegetables. And into the other plate he placed one stuffed green pepper, the rest of the fried potatoes, and a good serving of the mixed vegetables. Then, along with the cutlery and napkins, he served the halibut to Janice and put the plate with the stuffed pepper in front of his chair. He went back to the counter and brought out the serving platter filled with enough food for five people, and placed it in front of Karen.

Karen stared at the platter, looked at Fowler, then laughed.

Fowler said, "I thought you were starving?"

"I am."

"And you're always starving?"

"Yes!"

"Well, if you're always starving, you should be able to continually eat. So it seems to me I might even have to refill this platter. Maybe several times."

"Fowler," Karen said. "You're making fun of— "

"I understand starving," Fowler cut in. "I saw the movie. And I don't want that to happen here, not in front of me, not in my restaurant.

And so let's eat, because Janice and I are hungry. And I have another strategy to tell you about. Strategy number six. And if you thought drinking water was one of the easiest, then number six is definitely the hardest."

Karen sighed. First to Gabe she said, "They want to make me fatter — after I've just lost two and a half pounds." Then to Fowler she added, "But you know what? This smells too good to pass up. And at the moment I don't care about losing weight or gaining weight or anything else. I'm going to pretend that I'm alone, and just eat."

"We'll talk about that too," Fowler said, digging into his meal.

Karen said, "You know, this meatball—"

"Turkey," Janice said.

"Right, turkey, it's really unbelievable. I don't think I've ever tasted anything quite like it before."

"And you probably won't again," Janice said.

Karen, her mouth full, managed, "Why not?" She finished her turkey ball, took a bite of the eggplant parmesan, and said, "This is really excellent!"

"Do you remember what my father said about creativity and The Power of One?" Janice said. "That inside of it there are two types of creativity—the creativity he uses to tailor each of the strategies to his life, the way he did by putting lemon juice in his water or using the soy pepperoni for his pizza, or finding the fat or sugar in a meal and reducing it to as low as possible."

"That part's a game," Fowler said. "I still have fun with it."

"It's all a game to you," Janice said, turning to her father. "The entire Power of One. You have fun with all of it."

"You're right. I do have fun with it. I know I'm not supposed to, but I do. I like making it easy, making it... invisible. And I like the results."

Janice, still looking at her father, said, "You know, you shouldn't be saying that. According to all the overweight people out there, you're supposed to be struggling with this, moaning about all the good stuff you're not allowed to eat and how you'll never be able to make it last, not spending the last ten years having fun." She smiled and shook her head, then turned to Karen. "Where was I? Oh yes, creativity. There's the tailoring part of it, *making The Power of One easy*, even fun. Then there's this," she said, pointing to her vegetable rice. "The going-wild-in-the-kitchen side. And when it comes to this creativity, there's *less* to it than meets the eye."

"What do you mean?" Karen asked.

"What I mean is that if my father can cook like this, then anyone can. He might be a genius at taking nutritional complexities and reducing them into simple guidelines. But when it comes to cooking, to this part of it, the flavor part—"

"Okay, okay," Fowler said. "If we're going to air my dirty little secret, then at least let me do the airing." He looked at Karen. "It goes like this— there's a sale at the grocery store on green peppers, so, I buy a few..."

"Twenty," Janice said.

"Alright, twenty. Enough for the entire platoon. Then with all those green peppers I say, well, I just happen to have this defatted ground meat in the fridge."

"About a ton of it," Janice said. "*He likes to make his big batches of anything in stages, spread over a few days, so he doesn't really do very much at one time.*"

Fowler shrugged. "My concentration span is limited, and like everyone else, so is my time." Then he said, "Oh yes, the green peppers. So I snoop around the kitchen a bit more and I find some brown rice, maybe some onions, some vegetables, a few packages of frozen spinach, a dozen or so egg whites, the usual salt and pepper."

"But the flavor?" Karen said, thinking, *Spread out the work, that's an idea I can use.*

"The flavor," Fowler said, "is what I do when I've got the basics covered — I go for it." He grinned. "The flavor you're tasting now belongs to anything I might have had in the kitchen at the time I put those green peppers together. It could have been sage or curry powder or hot pepper flakes or thyme or ginger or a dozen other herbs or spices that at the moment sounded like they might blend well. Create cold fusion."

"You mean you don't remember?"

"Are you kidding? Of course not. And I don't care. If it's possible, I'll taste whatever I'm cooking while I'm cooking it. If not, if I'm spicing something raw, then I'll just play. Just have fun. And most of the time it works and some of the time it doesn't — and," he said, quickly turning to Janice with a raised warning finger, "I don't want to talk about any of my flavor disasters."

"Paprika on fried strawberries," Janice whispered.

"One strawberry! And it was a test."

"You see?" Janice said to Karen. "That's what I mean. His creativity in the kitchen is *nothing more than being fearless.*"

"Courage and creativity," Karen said.

Fowler nodded. "I've never met an herb or spice or vegetable I didn't invite into my kitchen at least once."

"But," Janice said, "don't let all this talk of creativity in the kitchen scare you. Because even for Fowler, who's definitely not a predictable kind of guy, a certain predictability does tend to develop. A sort of routine."

"Call it the house menu," Fowler said to Janice.

"I like that," Janice said. "The house menu." Then to Karen she said, "You see, even though he's always continually making something new, having fun, there's still the *core group of meals* that we always have on hand, meals that have become our *comfort foods,* meals that over time he's tailored to fit within the guidelines of the strategies, and learned to spice more or less consistently."

Fowler said, "Some of them I make on the spot, like all my breakfasts or my whole range of salads or my tuna specialties made with lemon juice and fat-reduced mayonnaise and Dijon mustard."

"He loves tuna packed in water," Janice said. "If he's in a hurry he'll just open a can, drain it, and eat it over the sink in about three minutes, and get back to whatever he's doing." She shook her head. "Another good example, though, of something he prepares on the spot, and one of my favorites, is his fettuccini alfredo made with one percent milk, cornstarch and soya parmesan cheese."

"Corn starch and just about any liquid makes a great gravy or sauce," Fowler said. "There's absolutely no need for butter. And that's a tip I got out of a low-fat cooking magazine. There's plenty of those out there — low-fat cooking magazines and books and internet sites and tv shows."

"And then for his lazy days," Janice continued, "for those times like now, when he doesn't want to cook anything, there's all those different items in the freezer, like the turkey balls you're eating, items that freeze well and store easily in his energy bank."

"And are ready in five minutes," Karen said. She turned to Fowler. "That's the part that's amazing. Not only have you figured out how to turn fat-filled meals that everyone loves into meals that are as low in fat as possible, but you've also developed this *system of beating being lazy, by being on top of things*, by keeping your freezer filled with delicious, throw-in-the-microwave-or-oven meals. You are one step ahead of the curve. When Gary and I aren't eating the garbage frozen meals that our freezer's filled with, we're ordering in." She smiled, then said, "What I'd like to do is order in from your freezer! This is so much better than the junk we have delivered. The junk we live on."

"That's what Janice is talking about," Fowler said, "the basic foods we live on. Our *comfort foods*. And that includes everything in my freezer. But I think it's that way with most families. Though certain foods — call them experimental foods or holiday foods — come and go, *there's a core set of foods, of meals, eight, ten, twelve, maybe, that are eaten over and over again — and each time fully enjoyed. The difference with me is that my core set of food is built around the strategies of The Power of One.*"

"And life goes on seamlessly," Janice said. "The Power of One goes to the core of our menu, takes over, and disappears."

Fowler broke the train of this conversation by saying, "We were supposed to be talking about the sixth strategy." Then he looked at Karen and her still mostly full plate, and said, "But before we do that, I want to know how you're doing with all that food. And even more importantly, I want to know if you're still starving."

CHAPTER
26

Karen looked into Fowler's eyes.

Once again Fowler said, "Are you still starving?"

Karen dropped her eyes to the food in her plate. She'd tasted each of the items, but had eaten only about twenty percent of the total amount, about as much food as Fowler had eaten. Left in Fowler's plate were just a couple of fried potatoes.

"The answer to the question isn't in the plate," Fowler said. "You're going to have to look somewhere else." He caught Janice's eye.

Janice said to Karen, "If you're not still starving, if you can't say that, then are you at least still hungry? The way I was hungry?"

Karen pressed her brows together. She had her fork in her hand with a turkey ball speared through it. She said, "This is really good food. I mean, *really* good."

Fowler laughed lightly. "That wasn't the question. The question was, are you still hungry? Is your stomach still telling you it *needs* food? You know, is it still growling? Still feeling sort of knotted? Is it still yelling its little stomach head off demanding food?" He waited a moment, got no response, then said once more, "I'm not going to tell you you have to stop eating. But just do this for me—put down your fork, take a good swallow of your water, and answer the question Are you still hungry?"

Karen did as Fowler asked. She placed her fork back onto her plate, took a swallow of her water, then said, "You know, the question

'Are you hungry?' is a question we get asked so often that we sort of forget it's a question. It's more of an invitation to eat. But once you start eating — once *I* start eating — there's never a point where I ask myself, Am I still hungry? Being not still hungry is not the reason for me to stop eating. That's not when I say, Okay, I've had enough. Being not hungry is not the trigger that gets me to put down my fork. Do you know what I mean?"

"I understand perfectly," Fowler said. "I was that way too. *Sometimes I still am.* Remember, I'm you. And being *not hungry*, having enough food in our stomachs so that it's stopped shouting for more, is *not* why we stop eating."

"You said that you're always starving," Janice said. "Can you think about that statement again? Can you still say you're always starving?"

Karen smiled. "That, at least, I can answer. And the answer is no. I'm not always starving. I mean, even though I said it and even meant it then, it's not true. How can anyone who eats regularly be always starving? Right now, I'm not starving. I'm not sure what I am. But I'm not starving. And with very little thought I can tell you there are times when I'm just the opposite of starving, when I'm stuffed."

"When you've swallowed the lead-filled beach ball," Janice said. "What?"

"The lead-filled beach ball. At least that's how Fowler describes it." She looked at her father and said, "He has a name for everything. And that's what he calls it when we eat so much we can barely move."

"Barely walk or talk or breathe," Fowler said. "When you have to stumble to a couch and collapse onto it and sit there with your belt open and legs spread and lower jaw hanging, sucking back air while this lead-filled beach ball you just forced down your gullet crushes you. And then you wait, and moan, and wait, until your body begins to digest some of it. Begins to give you some relief. It's completely ridiculous, but to differing degrees, that's what most of us call eating well. Satisfying our appetites. That's what I used to do." He laughed.

Karen didn't laugh with him. "You're describing me," she said. "I'll eat until I can't eat anymore. Until the plate's empty, no matter how much was on it, or until the baking dish is scraped clean or until the bag of chips is gone or until every container of the take-out food is picked through. I won't stop eating until there's nothing left to eat. *And it has nothing to do with still being hungry.* Of course I'm not still hungry. I'm stuffed. I've eaten the beach ball, and even then, if there's something else in the fridge or cupboard, some cookies or cake or ice cream or a piece of anything sweet left over from yesterday, I'll try to get that into my stomach too."

"I know what you're saying," Fowler said. "There was a time when food for me was an obsession. Stimulation. Adventure. Something to look forward to. Even plan for. But not in the way I look forward to or plan for now. It was much bigger then. Wide-screen. Technicolor.

"I used to think, Okay, tomorrow I'm going to buy that new book I've been wanting to read, and to make the reading of it better, more exciting, I'm going to get a double-size family pack of fried chicken and fries and the junk that comes with it, and read and eat for one, two, three hours, nonstop. And I would do just that! Slowly but steadily stuff myself until I was ready to burst. And then I'd feel sick, sometimes literally—and sometimes just about me, about how I could have done that." He shrugged. "I ate that way for years. Doubling your weight takes that kind of effort."

"I do the same thing," Karen said, "but I thought I was the only one."

Fowler shook his head. "You're not alone. You're the same as practically everyone out there who's lost control. We eat until we're stuffed, then watch tv, hit a commercial, maybe an ad for food, another cruise missile aimed into our homes, and eat some more. And on and on. And that behavior, that using food as a crutch, as entertainment, as stimulation, that eating until there's nothing left to eat, trying to satisfy yourself and never really doing it, isn't caused by The Enemy.

"But The Enemy does use it! We can feel it with every ad. They lock onto us with their big guns, their nuclear warheads, competing with each other to see who can kill us quickest with the largest servings or the thickest steak or the most selections in their all-you-can-eat fat factories. They know how our bodies work, they know our weaknesses, and they zero in on them, use them to seduce us into their arms, into their brightly colored, kid-friendly, plastic homes away from home, where they batter us and our children over and over by offering every kind of artery-clogging, obesity-creating food they can make a buck on!"

Fowler took a deep breath. "But the one thing The Enemy doesn't do is stand over us with a gun and say, Eat!"

"Can I blame him anyway?" Karen asked.

"You can blame anyone you want," Fowler said, "as long as you realize the solution to this particular problem is in here." He tapped his head. "You have to think it through. The key, just like the basic key to The Power of One, is knowledge. *Knowing what's behind your need to keep eating.* Understanding what your body's telling you. Listening to it *while you're eating.*"

"Let's start again," Janice said. She smiled at Karen, then once more asked, "Are you still hungry? Take your time. Talk to yourself. Think about it. If that feeling of being hungry is gone, and you still haven't stepped into lead-filled-beach-ball territory — then stop." Then she quickly said, "*But don't look for a feeling of being satisfied. That's not what I'm telling you to do.* I want you to look for a feeling of not needing to eat anymore. *Not needing to eat, starting to get full.* And if you have that feeling, then stop."

"Or take another bite," Fowler said. "But know that if you're not hungry anymore, if you've reached the point that Janice just described, of not feeling hungry, of starting to feel full, then know that that next bite is the one that'll cause your body to say to all its major parts, 'Hey, guys! Get ready! Because the boss is about to shove more food down her throat! Even though we already have plenty, more than enough to do our jobs, there's still more on the way! So everyone to your stations, because we're going to have to take that next bite and store it, just in case of famine, and for today we'll store it on her hips, and maybe tomorrow we'll pack it into a new chin.'"

"Stop eating," Janice urged.

"Take another bite," Fowler said. "Just one more. It's so good. Mmm mmm. Food. Tasty food."

Karen laughed. She shook her head and picked up her fork and looked at the turkey ball still on it and said, "You little devil! You tempting little devil!"

"Strategy number six," Fowler whispered. "Stop eating when you come to the point where you're not hungry anymore, where you're just beginning to feel full, and don't have even one more bite. No matter how much food is left on your plate, whether it's only a single turkey ball or still enough to feed an army, don't have even one more bite. And this is the hardest of the eight strategies to follow, the one that for me, at the beginning, took the greatest inner battle. But just like the other strategies, it got easier and easier with each new device I put into place to tailor it, to make it work for me, for my personality. Work to the degree I wanted it to work at the moment. In the situation."

"He got creative with it," Janice said. "And he had to, because with this strategy he's not fighting commonsense, he's fighting his genetics."

"I had to think it through," Fowler said. "Debate my genes. Use knowledge to fight instinct."

"What do you mean?" Karen asked.

Janice said, "The reason I said to stop eating when you feel *not* hungry, when you're just *starting to feel full*, and not when you feel satisfied, is because, genetically, *we're programmed to eat everything in front of us*. Genetically, we're not going to be satisfied until all the food on our plate is gone. That's why it's so easy to get into lead-filled-beach-ball territory. That's why it's so easy to use food as entertainment. It's part of our survival instinct. Eat all you can in case of famine."

"When it comes to eating," Fowler said, "feeling satisfied and being not hungry are two completely different things. Think about it. If you've got tempting food in front of you, like now, your body is screaming, 'Eat it! We don't know when we'll get this stuff again. Eat it, because we won't be satisfied until it's all gone!'

"But your body isn't saying, 'Eat it because we're still starving.' That feeling of starving is gone. And now you're trying to know if you even have the feeling of being hungry. And that's what you've got to pick out. And you've got to do it while your body is screaming, 'Eat the stuff so we can store it for the next big famine!'"

Janice smiled, but Karen wasn't smiling. She was staring at Fowler.

"One of the problems is that the food is *still there*," Fowler continued. "Still in front of you. That's the reason your body is still yelling. Because it can see it, smell it, still taste it on your taste buds. So your genetics, your instincts, all those parts, are continually yelling, 'Hey, good stuff! Eat! Eat! Keep on eating!'

"And so you can see why, with this strategy, with the concept of, 'Once I've got my hunger covered, I won't eat another bite,' my creativity had to begin with a lot of talking to myself. And that was forced on me by my genetics. Genetics forced me to talk to my head. Talk to my instincts. Talk to my courage. And then use my brains."

Janice was nodding.

Karen asked, "What did you say to yourself?"

"The first thing I said is what I already told you. I asked myself , Where, exactly, do I want that next bite of food to go? Back to my belly. To my thighs? To that roll I used to have under my chin? It's got to go somewhere, so I thought of where, and that pitted those guys yelling for more food against my mirror."

"Did that work?"

"Sometimes."

Karen laughed. But Fowler said, "I also told myself that what I had sitting on my plate in front of me was only food. It may have been great food, even exceptional food, but in the end, it's still only food, and there'll always be more. Another meal. And another. And another. Forever and ever until my last day. You see, what I was trying to do for my head was to put what was left in my plate into perspective, because there is no shortage of food, we'll never see that. Not even of the great stuff. We're never going to have a famine, not in this country. So I tried to tell that to my genetics. Sort of say to them, Calm down, guys. Relax. Quit taking your work so seriously."

"Did that work?"

"Sometimes."

This time it was Janice who laughed.

"Another device I used was to experiment with that last bite," Fowler said. "If I wasn't sure whether I'd reached the point of not being hungry, I'd take another bite, and wash it down with a good swallow of water. Then I'd think about how I was feeling, ask myself again, Are you still hungry? And if I still wasn't sure, I'd take another bite, and another good swallow of water, and I'd keep doing that, quietly, *working only with myself, with my head*, until I was sure that my feeling of hunger was gone. And being sure — at the beginning, at least — used to come only when I could already feel that I'd pushed myself into lead-filled-beach-ball territory. Then, of course, I'd get mad at myself. Yell at myself about those last bites, about which one of them wasn't necessary, and swear not to do it again. To be on top of it the next time."

"Did that work?"

"Sometimes." Fowler smiled. Janice also smiled. Fowler said, "What began to happen after a while, though, after a lot of talking back and forth with my head, was that I began to know, from growing experience, three things.

"First, I began to know what feeling not hungry felt like. It's a quiet, calm feeling, *approaching feeling full, but still a good distance away from feeling stuffed.* It's as though, if I could put it on a monitor, you know, like they have in hospitals, the line would be just slightly wavy. No big deal one way or the other. And I started to turn that feeling into one that said, I'm satisfied, because I'm not feeling hungry. So I can stop. No big deal. Just stop.

"And the second thing I began to know, which I learned over time, from experience, was *just how much to put into my plate.* And I began using that experience — preparing to stop before I started to eat. I would fill my plate with the amount I knew, from experience, I'd need to eat to not feel hungry, then bulk it up with salad to trick those guys downstairs into thinking that there was a ton of food on the plate and that the boss was going to eat it all. And I would. But we're talking a game here. With my head. And salad. Because the stuffed feeling you get from extra salad is not lead-filled-beach-ball territory. But you do feel full."

"You also experimented with plate sizes," Janice said. "Using smaller and smaller plates, and making them fuller and fuller."

Fowler laughed. "That's right. I'd forgotten about that." To Karen he said, "When I first began to focus on this strategy, I did whatever I could, whatever I had to, because I knew that my genetics were not going to put up a fair fight."

Janice said, "Tell her the third thing you learned."

"The third thing I learned, from experience, from really focusing on this strategy and on myself and this business of eating, and stopping eating, was that though it seemed hard to stand up, leave the table, stop putting food into my mouth, if I did it — if I left the table and went on with whatever else I had to do, even putting the food and dishes away — *that feeling of needing to eat more disappeared.* In seconds. Because it's *not a true feeling.* I mean, I know I could still have pushed down two or three more meals if I let myself, but that strong urge was gone. For then at least. Until the next time I legitimately felt hungry."

Karen nodded. "You did what you could to either keep temptation away — or take it away."

"That's exactly it! That became *my most important life adjustment* to this strategy. *I kept, and I keep, temptation away.* I work at creating a situation where it's *easy* to say, That was good. I'm not hungry anymore. I know I can still shove a lot more food down, but I don't have it in front of me — so I won't.

"And after a while it became easy. Much easier than I could have imagined, because most of what we eat are foods we eat over and over again, so from experience, I just know how much is enough. And that's the strongest tool I rely on. *Using the knowledge of how much is enough has become second nature, a habit.* Using that knowledge has made this strategy, like all the others, become an invisible part of my life. I just do it now. There's no more great debate, no diet mentality, no worrying about being perfect, and no guilt about being human."

"Tell her about your pizza," Janice said.

"The pizza's a perfect example because I love it. And I eat it a lot. But when I eat it, I'll only serve myself two slices. It started out being four, then three, but now it's only two, because now I know that two slices of the size pizza I make, along with a salad, is all I need to eat to be able to say, That's it, the hunger's gone, I'm approaching feeling full, but still not even close to feeling stuffed.

"And I also know that the rest of the pizza is still close at hand. No one is going to steal it from the fridge. It can be eaten at the next snack, or the next meal, or the next day. Or made again, and again. Or replaced with something else.

"And," Fowler said, "you can always do this." He lifted his napkin, unfolded it, and gently placed it over the remaining fried potatoes in his plate. "There," he said. "Out of sight. Out of mind. Then," he added, smiling, "there's also this device." He stood, went to the fridge, and came back with a bowl of fruit.

"I thought of this one," Janice said.

Fowler picked an apple out of the bowl, tossed it into the air, caught it, and took a bite, then said, "Janice taught me to change the taste in my mouth. Take away the yummy taste of the spuds or the pizza or whatever I'd been eating, by having a fruit—Mother Nature's own dessert."

Karen, nodding, said, "The key here, the same as with the other strategies, is to think ahead. Work with yourself until you know the right amount of food for you, then serve yourself only that amount. Then walk away, knowing there's always the next snack or meal." She pressed her lips to a determined line, pushed the platter of food to the center of the table, and reached for an orange. And smiled at Fowler.

Fowler said, "Exactly."

Janice looked at Fowler. "After learning this strategy — to stop eating when you're no longer hungry and not take another bite—after you figured out the way to do that and make it a part of your life, The Power of One seemed to take over. It was at this point that you stopped working at it and simply let it sweep you away."

"I remember that," Fowler said. "I hit a kind of critical mass. But it was really a culmination of the strategies I knew up to then." To Karen he said, "I was already letting the excitement of any result I got from the strategies push me forward. But by this strategy, by the time I'd tailored this one so completely into my life that it disappeared, the effect of The Power of One had become... overwhelming."

In a whisper, Karen said, "I've just barely begun applying any of what I know so far, but I've also begun to see results. And I'm also beginning to feel something."

"That's exactly what I want," Fowler said. "But I don't want you to rush it. *Don't push The Power of One. Let it push you.* Take one tiny step, only one, then look around, see what you see, feel what you feel, *know that that single step is a great success in itself.* And then, when you're ready, take another step, and then another, and never let yourself fall into the *diet mentality trap.* Never let any of it make you anxious or worried or feeling guilty. Never."

"I'm ready for that now," Karen said. "What I'm feeling now is excitement. An expectation of something good about to happen." She paused for a moment and smiled. "And I'm planning on making a lot of that happen tomorrow night."

"You sound as though you're about to fly off on your honeymoon," Janice said.

"I do, don't I?" Karen laughed. "It's because that's what I'm feeling. That kind of excitement. And Gary doesn't know anything about it. I have the whole evening planned as a surprise. A fantasy evening for the two of us. One that includes The Power of One." She sighed. "He is my first priority. Him and Gabe. And I'm going to make it work. I'm going to make all of it work."

CHAPTER
27

"There. That's finished," Karen said, looking around the room with a sense of satisfaction. She walked over to Gabe's playpen, lifted him up, and gave him a hug.

She'd begun first thing in the morning, the moment Gary left for work, a room-by-room, corner-by-corner scrubbing. Now the town-house was immaculate—and she knew she was one step closer to her goal of a total change. A change in herself. A change in her marriage. A change in her life's priorities. Whether you know it or not, Gary, she said to herself, hugging Gabe once more, things are going to get better.

He hadn't kissed her before he left for work, he hadn't done that since the first year of their marriage, but he had looked at her, given her what she thought was something close to a smile—an indication, at least, that the transformation he'd begun seeing in her this past week was starting to have an effect on him.

And that look, no matter how small and quick, had had an effect on her. She'd wanted to run after him when he'd closed the door, reach him before he got to the car, tell him she knew it was going to work —be good again, fresh and vibrant and loving and caring, the way it had been at the beginning. And that she was going to lose the weight —especially that, lose all the weight The Enemy had seduced her into gaining, become finally, and this time permanently, the woman he'd married.

But she hadn't run after him because she knew words were too easy to say, that she'd said them too often in the past. And those easy words usually produced a sarcastic, cutting response. This time, she decided, she was going to save her words — and show him instead.

She carried Gabe into the kitchen, placed him into the high chair, and gave him his colored rings to play with. The radio was on loud and she began to sing along with it, thinking, Time to begin, to create *my own* Power of One restaurant, to break down the strategies into a form *I* can accept. Tailor them, the way Fowler taught me, *to fit Gary's life and mine.*

As little fat as possible, she'd written in her journal. Now she was on a hunt for fat.

She still had to accommodate Gary, she knew. That was important. And herself too. She had to be aware of their own comfort level. She would begin slowly, the way Fowler had begun, let her involvement in The Power of One *build of its own momentum,* be result-driven and not forced. This was not a diet. It required courage, some courage, and thought and planning and choices — *but no pain or sacrifice or any part of a diet mentality.*

And since Gary left the food shopping and cooking — and virtually the kitchen itself — to her, the process of defatting, of creating her Power of One haven, was hers alone. And she was glad for that.

She began with the obvious, replacing the butter and margarine and oil, except for one small jar of olive oil, with cans of nonstick spray. She smiled to herself, thinking she must have looked odd going through the checkout counter at the grocery store with half a dozen cans of just that item. But she'd been pleased to find that the sprays came in different flavors — butter and olive oil and one spiced with lemon. She hadn't known that. And those flavors, she knew, would make it impossible for Gary to tell the difference between her new method of cooking and the old.

To go with the nonstick spray she'd also bought several nonstick pans—three frying pans of differing sizes, two sauce pans, and two baking trays. They were less expensive than she'd imagined and were now the only way she would cook. In her journal she wrote, *Unless it's broiled, boiled, steamed, or cooked on the outdoor grill, it'll be prepared in a nonstick pan without fat!*

It was a good start, she knew, one that on its own would produce results. But she'd gone even further, replacing all the dairy products she used with similar items—but only those marked fat-reduced. She realized, however, that though these initial steps were very positive, they were still the easy part of the battle to find and eliminate fat, just scratching the surface. The real battle was in the cooking itself, in her choice of foods and the preparation. But just like Fowler, she knew she could do it. She would use her commonsense and creativity to incrementally, and continuously, for the rest of her life, gain health for herself and her family.

"Okay," she said to herself. "What's next?"

She went to the fridge, opened the door, and stared. Then took out the peanut butter and mayonnaise. "I love you guys," she said, holding up the two jars. "But I know there's a fat-reduced version of you somewhere, or else a *perfectly acceptable replacement*, and so you're history." She tossed them into the garbage and laughed, then opened the door to the freezer and reached for the icecream, but quickly pulled back her hand. In a conspiratorial whisper she said to the frozen bucket, "You can stay there for now, but you'd better keep your nose clean, mister, because you are definitely on probation."

She closed the freezer door, reached for her glass of lemon-flavored water and took a good swallow. She'd emptied one pitcher already today, and though she wasn't counting glasses, she was aware of her need to drink.

From yesterday to this morning she'd lost another half pound and she knew she hadn't yet put even a fraction of what she was planning into effect. All she had done so far was focus on the water, on using mostly egg whites and hardly any yolks, on eating breakfast, and on not buying the donut in the morning that had become her habit, replacing it instead with whole-wheat toast and fat-reduced cream cheese. She might have been satisfied with just that, she knew. Three pounds in six days with virtually no effort was just about miraculous. But that loss of three pounds was now pushing her. Fowler was right. Results produced excitement, and excitement created an urge to get even greater results. And this urge became the push for her to find even more ways to apply the six strategies she'd learned so far.

Yesterday, as she was leaving Fowler's house, she'd asked him to tell her what the last two strategies were, but he said he wanted to wait until she had more time. "Work with what you already have," he'd said. "The last two are beauties. You're going to love them both. And I don't want to just hand them to you. I want to gift-wrap them first, present them as the prizes they are." He'd laughed at her curiosity. So had Janice.

Well, I will work with what I have so far, she thought.

Tonight would be the first as-low-in-fat-as-possible meal for her and Gary. It would be as-low-in-sugar-as-possible too. And no part of it would be a made-in-a-factory meal. And for her, it would also be a meal where she was going to serve herself only the amount she thought would take away her hunger — that, and a hefty salad with fat-reduced dressing. And if she felt she was *approaching being full* before she'd eaten everything in the plate, she'd stop eating. Stop then, at that moment, and not have even one more bite.

From this point on, her life was going to be different. She had her priorities now. And she was one of them.

She glanced at the clock. Although there was still plenty of time, she wanted to begin preparing the meal early, allow herself room to experiment. "Courage and creativity," she said. "Those are my defenses. And the strategies are my weapons."

She'd thought out the menu and the evening carefully.

What she was hoping for tonight was simply that Gary realize she was there. That she existed. She envisioned them eating the meal together in the dining room, with Gabe in his high chair between them. The stereo would be playing softly and the television would be off. She was going to use the good dishes, light the fancy candles. She wanted to create a warm atmosphere. Most of all, though, what she wanted was to talk.

Just talk.

About anything.

It had been so long since Gary had told her how his day had gone, who'd done what or said what. It had been so long since he'd sighed and leaned back in his chair with his hands crossed behind his head and told her one of the dreams he had for their future — the cottage in the country, time to go fishing. Time to be together.

She wanted to see him smile. Hear him laugh. Watch him once again become the man she had married. The man with the quick sense of humor, with shoulders she could lean on. The man who was caring with her, conscious of her needs. The man she had fallen in love with.

"We can do it, Gary," she whispered. "*I* can do it. I know I can. With Fowler's help, with The Power of One, I'll change. You'll see."

She kissed Gabe on the forehead, rattled his rings, offered him a cookie, then picked it up off the floor when he said no.

The menu she'd planned was quick and easy. Keep it simple, she'd told herself while shopping. Let this meal become one of our *core meals*, replacing one of the core meals we live on now, any one of those high-fat mistakes, the burgers and french fries, or fried chicken with gravy, or ordered-in pizza or Chinese. Let it become a new staple, a new *comfort food.*

She took six skinless chicken breasts from the fridge and removed all the visible fat and cleaned them.

Gary, she knew, could eat two. She would eat one, and then see. And the other three would go into her energy bank. She smiled. She was starting an *energy account.* She would make her first deposit tonight and begin to build up her capital. She already thought it would be a good idea to buy another freezer, a small one that fit unobtrusively into a corner, and fill it with meals and snacks the way Fowler had, for those times when her energy was simply not there. She would not let the excuse of fatigue interfere with her progress. She would not let *any excuse* break her stride.

Hold on there, girl, she thought. One thing at a time. I have to let The Power of One work for me! I have to let the excitement it creates push me forward until an extra freezer becomes a matter of course, like breathing, like taking each of the strategies to the greatest degree my comfort level allows *without falling into the diet-mentality trap.* I have to let the force of The Power of One build until it becomes so ingrained in my life it becomes... invisible.

And it'll happen! It will! The same way it had for Fowler. And it'll work for Gary too, even if he won't know what's happening until he begins to see his own results. She laughed, picturing Gary's face when she eventually told him why they were both losing weight and gaining health, knowing that something as positive as The Power of One's strategies could not get a negative reaction, not even from him. What had Fowler said? *It's hard to argue about something that feels good.* Well, losing weight and gaining health were certainly going to feel good!

"Seamlessly," she whispered. That's how it works for Fowler and Janice, and that's how it's going to work for us. There's no apparent difference in the way they live now and the way they lived before The Power of One. No apparent difference — except that Fowler lost enough weight to build his own twin!

Okay, she thought, placing the cleaned chicken breasts aside. Get creative, get the juices flowing. I'm serving two very important guests tonight, VIPs of the highest order — my husband and me!

CHAPTER
28

Karen's first thought was to make the crunchy potatoes that Fowler loved. It would be a perfect replacement for the fat-filled french fries that Gary could eat seven nights a week. But then she decided to try something different.

One of Gary's favorite dishes, she knew, was scalloped potatoes. For him it was a comfort food from years ago, a dish his grandmother used to make for him and his brother. The only thing was that his grandmother, then his mother and me, Karen thought, used butter and fat-filled cheddar cheese and whole milk to prepare it. "That's just not acceptable anymore," she said aloud. "Think, girl. You can do this."

She began by peeling, then thinly slicing, the potatoes and a couple of onions. Then, instead of buttering her baking dish the way she normally would, she sprayed it with the nonstick spray. Next she layered about a third of the potatoes into the dish, and over this spread the sliced onion, a sprinkle of flour, salt and pepper, and a good handful of grated fat-reduced cheddar cheese.

"Looking good," she said, as she repeated the process, adding a second layer of potatoes to the pan. Then she went to the fridge and took out the one percent milk that only yesterday would have been fat-laden whole milk. After heating the milk in a sauce pan, she poured it over the potatoes, finishing the dish by sprinkling more fat-reduced cheddar over all and topping the cheddar with a Fowler-like flourish of dried parsley.

"You," she said to herself, carrying the baking dish to the oven, "are one creative genius!" Then she laughed, knowing the process of turning a fat-filled meal into one that had as little fat as possible was so simple that even Gabe, if he could read, if he could stand, would have been able to do it. Anyone could do it, she thought — if they knew the words to the first strategy. As low in fat as possible. Change the butter to the spray. The whole milk to one percent. The cheese to fat-reduced. It was just a matter of choices. Of preparing in advance to have those items on hand. Of creating a fat-reduced haven. "Thank you, Fowler," she said, before turning to the chicken.

The chicken recipe she was about to make had no name, because she was planning to make it up as she went along. Be creative, she thought. Tailor it to The Power of One and the customer's needs.

Gary liked onions and mushrooms, especially together, so she began with that.

She diced two large onions and placed them and an entire package of sliced mushrooms into a frying pan coated with the butter-flavored nonstick spray. Then she went to the cupboard where she kept her spices.

She was looking for tarragon, a spice she knew she had, but had never used. Fowler had said to be fearless, she thought. Well, she was planning on being even more than fearless tonight. She was going to be Fowler!

The tarragon was only the start.

She went back to the fridge and took out a bottle of white wine that had been sitting behind Gabe's apple juice for weeks.

Okay, she thought. Tarragon. Wine. Salt. Pepper. Maybe something with a bit of a tang. Like lemon juice!

"Go for it, Martha Stewart!" she said, snapping her fingers, finding the lemon in the refrigerator drawer.

She placed the chicken breasts into the pan with the nicely cooking onions and mushrooms, added the salt and pepper and tarragon, and atop it all, a good squeeze of the lemon, then with a brave "I hope this works," poured in a cup or so of the wine.

The radio was blaring. Her hips were swaying. She played a funky little beat with her wooden spoon against the side of the frying pan.

Then she thought, Veggies, not needing to refer to her notes to remember that Fowler had talked about a reasonable portion of as-low-in-fat-as-possible protein, alongside a potato or pasta or rice dish, and then a deeply colored vegetable or two, and the salad. The natural order of our meals, he called it. Well-rounded and well-balanced, tasty and satisfying — *the exact opposite of gimmicky fad diets designed to twist your head into a knot and your willpower into a pretzel.*

She went to the freezer, took out a package of frozen asparagus and got them steaming. Then did the same to a package of baby carrots — both packages free of oil, butter or sauce. Then she opened a bag of fresh salad, poured it into a bowl, added a dash of fat-reduced dressing, and said aloud, "Girl, you've done it! One unbelievable Power of One meal — in practically no time at all!"

She suddenly felt like celebrating, then realized, It's not the effort, that's not the reason to celebrate. *Because there was no effort. None beyond what I would usually have spent to make any meal.* It's the fact that this meal will add to Gary's health and mine. That this meal, which is actually two meals, because I made enough to bank both the chicken and the potatoes in the freezer, will cause us to lose weight.

"We have to eat to lose weight," she said, repeating what Fowler had told her. You were right, Fowler. It's the knowledge that's powerful. It's the knowledge that's going to change my life and turn me into half the woman I am now!

And I can hardly wait!

When the chicken was ready, she put it into a nonstick baking dish to be kept warm in the oven alongside the scalloped potatoes and asparagus and baby carrots tossed in the butter-flavored nonstick spray. Then she prepared the dining room table with the good dishes and two candles, changed the music from the radio to a cd, and took her shower.

By the time she heard Gary open the front door, she was dressed, had put on makeup and a hint of perfume, had just finished changing Gabe, and was now placing him into his high chair at the dining room table.

Gary first walked into the kitchen, then the dining room.

Karen, in a soft hopeful voice, said, "Hi."

"What's going on?" Gary wanted to know.

"Nothing's going on," Karen said. "I just thought we'd do something different tonight."

Gary looked at the table, at the setting, the candles, then at Karen. His initial expression seemed bewildered. Then that changed to something closer to amusement.

Karen smiled.

But Gary's amusement lasted only seconds. He said, "You're ridiculous. You're fat and stupid and ridiculous." And with that he turned and left the room and in a moment slammed the front door to the town-house. Even from the dining room, Karen could hear him screech the tires on his car.

For one long minute, then two, then five, Karen did not move. Her expression, too, remained blank. Then she said to Gabe, "It's alright. It's just the first try. It took time for it to get bad, and it'll take a bit of time for it to get good again. But it will. You'll see, it will."

Then she stood, walked to the kitchen, took out the pan of scalloped potatoes and the one filled with the chicken breasts and the third with the asparagus and baby carrots, and very calmly scraped all three pans into the garbage. Then she went to the drawer, took out a spoon, went to the freezer, took out the ice cream, and walked back to the dining room.

CHAPTER
29

Karen, with Gabe in her arms, stood on Fowler's back porch. She could hear Fowler's voice, though his words were muffled, coming from somewhere inside the house. Then she heard Janice clearly saying, "I can't!"

For a moment Karen hesitated, unsure whether to stay or return home. Then she forced herself to knock. Courage's welcoming bark brought an agitated Fowler to the door.

It had been ten days since she was last here and declared she was now her own person, able to choose her own friends, decide whether or not The Power of One was for her. Ten days since she'd vowed to fight for her health and her marriage.

And she'd fought.

And Gary'd fought back.

First by ridiculing her efforts, her weight, her intelligence, then by shutting her out of his life through a silent treatment so complete it virtually paralyzed her, left her able to make only a couple of short, teary calls to Janice. Then none at all. Then last night Gary had come home at three in the morning and told her to get out of his bed, that he wouldn't sleep with her anymore, and that from now on she could sleep on the couch.

After Gary left for work, Karen took the shortcut through the woods to Fowler and Janice's house. She was struggling with another morning-after-the-fight daze. But this time, she knew, things were different. This time she had no fight left in her. She was tired.

Emotionally battered and drained. And this time, too, she weighed more than when she'd last been here. I'm numb, she thought. Resigned to whatever Gary wants to throw at me. I've gone beyond hopelessness. There's nothing left. No courage. None.

But this morning Karen found the mood tense at Janice and Fowler's.

From behind the counter Fowler asked, "What can I get you for breakfast?" He wore a troubled expression and there were no pleasantries from him, not for Karen or Janice.

At the table, Janice had an untouched cup of tea in front of her and nothing else. No books. No papers. No magazines. Even the newspaper she usually read lay unopened.

Though the baby seat was still in its place, Karen sat at the table with Gabe in her arms. She wasn't going to eat here, she decided. Nor was she going to learn the rest of The Power of One. Coming here had been a mistake. She was going to go home, rewind the tape of her marriage, and keep playing it over. She said to Fowler, "Nothing. Not today. I won't be having breakfast."

Janice looked at Karen. "Breakfast is one of the strategies."

Karen shook her head. "I have no strategies."

Fowler stepped past the counter to the table but didn't take his seat. He simply looked at Karen.

Dropping her eyes, Karen said, "I'm sorry. I know you don't want to hear this. But there are no strategies for me. Not anymore. Not for me."

"If there are no strategies," Janice asked, "then what is there?"

For a moment Fowler stood with his arms crossed over his chest, expression grim. Then he suddenly clapped his hands and said loudly, "What there is, is breakfast out! At someone else's restaurant. With someone else's food. And it's on me. And we're going now!"

Janice turned her head to Fowler and looked at him as though he'd just spoken a strange language.

"Now!" Fowler said. "I mean it. The day is young and I feel great and I want to get going." He stared into Janice's eyes.

Janice began to say, "I'll wait for you—"

"You're not waiting anywhere," Fowler interrupted. "I said *we're* going out. The four of us. And you have five minutes to get ready. Or I'm going to put on my khaki shorts with my cowboy boots and miner's lamp, and if you think one unusually shaped woman with a beautiful smile, one slightly overweight woman who's lost her strategies, and one perfect little boy are a sight, you're going to have to live with that too." He didn't laugh.

Neither did Janice or Karen.

Janice said, "I can't."

Fowler said, "You can." He turned to Karen. "Other than going to the hospital, Janice has never left this house. Not once in twenty-six years. I'm to blame for some of that time. But not all of it."

Again Janice whispered, "I can't. I'm sorry. I can't face other people." She turned to Karen and began to say, "I'm a freak—"

"No!" Karen cried, and sat upright as though she'd been jolted with an electric shock.

"It's the truth," Janice said. "You don't see it anymore. But I am a freak. Nothing but a—"

"Stop saying that!" Karen shouted, suddenly breaking into tears. She reached for Janice's hand and held it tightly. Courage stood.

Fowler said, "We talked about courage and creativity. We talked about The Power of One. We talked about priorities. But what we haven't talked about are *walls*. Getting through the walls *we're all inevitably going to find in our way*, the walls blocking our chosen path, holding us back."

Weeping softly, Karen said, "How do we get through those walls? What's the answer?"

"The only way to get through any wall," Fowler said, "is to do it. Confront the wall. Do what needs to be done. And take it down."

CHAPTER

30

Karen got into the back seat with Gabe while Fowler helped Janice into the front. He folded Janice's portable wheelchair and placed it in the car's trunk. Courage, nose against the living room window, barked anxiously.

Karen's eyes were moist.

Janice wept quietly. She'd first said no, then yes, then no again, then changed her mind one last time to a final yes — and stuck to it. "But I'm afraid," she whispered then, "more afraid than I've ever been in my life."

Fowler, putting the car into drive, said, "Boy, talk about your happy outings."

Fowler waited in front of Karen's town-house while Karen got Gabe's car seat from her own car. She snapped the seat into the back seat of Fowler's and adjusted Gabe securely. Although there was no one about on the street, Janice hunched down in the front seat.

Fifteen minutes later Fowler pulled into the handicap parking spot in front of the restaurant, got the wheelchair, and lifted Janice from the car to the chair, covering her lap and legs with the blanket.

"Please stay close to me," Janice said to Karen.

Karen, with Gabe in her arms, answered, "I'm right here. I'll be right beside you the whole time."

Fowler guided Janice's wheelchair to the access ramp and up and through the automatic doors, where they were met by the hostess.

"Hello," she said. "Will that be four?" Then she looked at Janice and her smile died. She snapped her eyes away, looked back again, then focused wide-eyed on Fowler's hard expression.

It was Karen who said, "Yes, four, and we'll need a high-chair for the baby."

Janice's eyes remained lowered.

The hostess, a pretty woman in her twenties, replied, "Oh yes. Of course." She showed them to a corner table where she cleared a place for the wheelchair while studiously avoiding even another glance at Janice.

Fowler moved Janice to the table. The hostess left, then quickly returned with the high-chair and three menus. She placed the menus onto the table and said, "Your waitress will be with you in just a few minutes. Enjoy your meal."

"Thank you," Fowler said.

Karen seated herself next to Janice.

Janice's eyes were still cast low. She reached for her menu but did not open it. In a whisper she said to Karen, "Is anyone looking?"

Karen turned toward the other customers in the restaurant.

Many eyes were on Janice, some discreetly, and others less so. For a moment Karen too dropped her head, only to look up into Fowler's angry expression.

Fowler said to her, "She asked you a question and I think she deserves an answer."

Karen turned to Janice. "Yes," she said, "some people are looking." Once again she put her hand on Janice's shoulder.

Janice was trembling. She lowered her head even further and whispered, "Help me."

The waitress stepped up to the table with three coffees and placed them, saying, "Are you ready to order yet?" Karen could tell she had been briefed by the hostess because she did not look at Janice.

"No," Karen answered. "We'll need a few more minutes."

"Sure thing," the waitress said, stepping away.

Janice said, "I have to leave."

Fowler was staring at her.

"But we're already here," Karen said. "The hardest part is over. You took the first step. Found the courage to do that. For the first time in your life you left your house to go someplace other than the hospital, knowing what to expect. And now you're here, at your wall." She paused for a moment, then in a low voice said, "Confront it, Janice. Do what Fowler said. Face it. Take down your wall."

Again Karen looked at Fowler. His expression remained hard, but he was nodding. Suddenly she realized that what she'd just done for Janice was describe The Power of One, though this time without relating it to nutrition. In exactly the same way that being overweight controls my life, she thought, Janice's fear controls hers. And the process to overcome both are the same. *Find the courage, go with the knowledge, take that first step, and then confront any wall that gets in the way.*

Janice, her head still bowed, voice slow and filled with pain, said, "You don't know what it feels like. You can't."

"What does it feel like?" Fowler said. "Tell us."

"It feels like I'm on display," Janice quickly answered, her voice breaking now. "Like I'm a sideshow—"

Karen touched Janice's hand, the gesture a plea for her to not use the word *freak*. Janice said nothing further.

"No," Fowler said. "Not that. We already know that, and we understand. And you're right. To a certain extent you are on display, for a little while at least. You look different from the rest of us. You have a disability. And people are curious. We know all that. We came in here knowing that, knowing what to expect, and now you've hit a difficult moment. You're at your wall. And I want to know what that feels like. That part that only you can feel."

Janice lifted her head slightly and looked at Fowler. "What do you mean?"

"I mean, what does it feel like to be at your wall? What does it feel like to be in the process, right now, as we speak, of breaking through your wall? I want to know what you're feeling now, at this exact moment." His voice had begun to rise. His expression was growing harsher. When the waitress walked up he waved her off with a curt "Not yet!"

Janice continued to stare into Fowler's eyes. It took her a moment before she said, speaking very slowly, "It feels as though I'm being eaten alive. As though all of my muscles are screaming, just screaming with pain. As though I'm forcing myself through a vat of thick, heavy acid. Burning acid. This process is slow, and painful, and every ounce of my being is crying out to not be here. I don't want to be here. I don't want the pain. I want to go home." She closed her eyes, let the tears fall. Then opened her eyes abruptly and said, her voice too beginning to rise, "But I have no choice, do I? I can't just leave on my own. I'm here because I'm being forced to be here."

For a moment Fowler said nothing. Then he said, staring directly into Janice's eyes, "You do have a choice. Say it again. Tell me once more that you want to leave and I'll take you home. Take you out of this... process. This effort. Take you back to what you know, to where you can draw the curtains again and hide. Say it one more time — 'I want to leave.'"

Janice stared at her father.

"Say it now!" Fowler said.

Karen, thrusting out a suddenly clenched fist, said to him, "Don't you — !"

But Fowler cut her off with, "You stay out of this! What do you know about what's happening here? There's no one, no one in this room, who has half the courage Janice has. No one! Only she doesn't know it. Not yet. She doesn't know that for twenty-six years I've looked to her to find my strength. That I've looked to her to get the strength I needed to be able to do the little I've done with my life!"

"I'll stay," Janice said suddenly.

Fowler turned to her. "Are you sure?"

"Yes, I don't want to go back. I'll go through the pain. I'll get through it. I don't want to go back. It's time to stop hiding." She stared at Fowler.

Karen's eyes filled with tears.

Fowler said to Janice, "I love you."

"I know."

"I'm sorry."

"I'm not," Janice said. "I'm glad it happened." She lifted her head a little higher, turned it slightly toward Karen, and said, "Thank you."

Karen nodded, then looked at Fowler and, after a long pause, said, "We all have our walls, don't we?"

"Yes," Fowler answered. "We all have our walls. In that way, we're all alike. The only difference is in how we handle our walls when we get to them."

Again, for a long moment no one spoke. Karen knew that Fowler and Janice, like her, were taking in the enormity of what had just happened. Finally Karen said to Fowler, "An hour ago I told you I had no strategies. I had come to my wall. I let it stop me. But now I want my strategies back. I'm ready to break through my wall." She reached for Janice's hand.

CHAPTER

31

"Then take your strategies back," Fowler said to Karen.

"Just like that?"

"Yes. Just like that. They're yours to take. They're a part of you now. And a part of the process of owning The Power of One is using it, and walking away from it, and going back again, as many times as you have to."

"Is that what happened to you?"

"*That's what still happens.* There's no end to walls, to situations. We do our best. And at times our best isn't good enough and we fall back on old ways. And then, when we can, we pick ourselves up and crash through the wall that jumped into our path and move on, *knowing other walls will come up.* Walls that we'll handle as we get to them." He shook his head. "This is real life, Karen, not playtime. *Diets are playtime.* You go to the playground, play the diet, struggle under the diet mentality, then go home—go back to real life. The Power of One is real life. It's part of the package. And real life isn't always pretty. We fall down and scrape our knees. Then get back up and move on. And The Power of One moves on with us — continues to move on — for the rest of our lives." He met Janice's eyes and smiled at her.

"So I can try again?" Karen said.

"No," Fowler said, turning back to Karen. "You can *do it* again."

Karen stared at him, then took a deep breath and, in a determined voice, said, "Then the strategies are again mine. I reclaim them."

"Good. That's what I wanted to hear."

"All six of them."

Fowler grinned. "Do you remember that I told you the last two strategies were gifts?"

"Of course I remember. And I've wanted to know what you meant by that since you said it. How could something you're supposed to do when it comes to eating be considered a gift?"

"They are gifts. Believe me." Fowler glanced again at Janice. Her head was fully raised now and she was slowly, cautiously, looking about the room. He reached across the table and pressed his fingers around hers. "Are you okay?"

Janice nodded.

He squeezed her hand once more, then leaned back in his seat and cleared the emotion from his throat. "What's the best thing about eating?" he asked Karen.

"The best thing about eating, is just... eating."

"That's right," Fowler said.

"It is?"

"Of course it is. The best thing about eating is eating. I love to eat. You love to eat. Everyone loves to eat. And the reason *strategy number seven* is a gift is because it says just that, Eat often."

"Eat often? How can that be?"

"The human body wasn't designed to survive on just three meals a day," Fowler said. "That's a rule society came up with. And it's a rule we can ignore. What we really want to do is eat five or six times a day. Every two or two and a half or three hours. Whatever's convenient. However the strategy will be tailored to suit your needs at the time."

"Eat five or six times a day?"

"That's right. Remember when we invited you for lunch and you said you were starving? And Janice and I said we were hungry, but not starving. Well that's one of the problems with eating only three times a day. We get too hungry between meals — then we stuff ourselves."

"The lead-filled beach ball."

"Exactly. What we want to do is eat often and follow all the other strategies —"

"To the degree we're comfortable with them," Karen said.

Fowler nodded. "Let's go back to my car analogy. What I want to do is change that clunker into a sports car, a sleek, healthy Ferrari. And since I have to start somewhere, the first thing I'm going to change is the gas tank. And I'm doing this to make room for that muscular engine that's still on order. So I put in a sports-car gas tank, a much smaller tank than the one it has now. And because of the smaller tank, I have to refill it more often. So, for example, I'll eat a meal..."

"Breakfast."

"Breakfast. Then go on a short trip, to the garden, the computer, the grocery store, then two or three hours later, I'll eat again. Refill the tank. And the food I eat can be anything — so long as it falls into the guidelines of the other strategies. It can be another meal or a snack or yesterday's leftovers. Anything.

"And I'm off again. On another trip, and this one will take me to noon or so, and then I'll —"

"Eat again," Karen said. "And again and again and again. I can do that. I want to do that!"

Fowler said, "We're building our sports car from the inside out — by each time filling the tank with only the right amount of the right kind of fuel. *Just the right amount and the right kind of food to get us to the next fill-up.* To get us from mildly hungry, to not hungry, to mildly hungry again, as often as we need. And this also keeps our blood-sugar levels *naturally stable*, knocking down a whole slew of fad diet myths that focus on that. And we do all of this within our personally tailored strategic limits. All within the limits we can each live with." He grinned, then asked, "Would you call this strategy a gift?"

"This strategy," Karen said, "is the best gift I've had in a long, long time. Permission to eat whenever I'm hungry."

CHAPTER

32

The waitress, this time from a distance, said, "Excuse me. Everyone here okay with ordering now?"

"Just a few more minutes," Fowler said. He turned to Janice. "What would you like to eat?"

Though the menu was in front of her, Janice still hadn't opened it. "Do they have pancakes?" she asked. "I'll have that."

Fowler now looked at Karen. Her menu was open, but she said, "I don't know what to choose. I mean, I'm not... I haven't..."

Glancing at his own menu, Fowler said, "The pancakes are a good choice, if you stay away from the butter and be careful with the syrup. So is the fruit cup." He leaned closer to Karen. "When we go out to eat there are really only three things we need to be aware of. The first is the fat. *These places simply don't work with our first strategy*, so you can count on most of the items on their menu being loaded with fat. And the *second is the sugar* — though the sugar is more easily controlled.

"And the third is the *size of the servings*, because the least expensive part of running a restaurant is the cost of the food. So they use the size of the servings as a lure to get us in. But there are ways around each of these problems. First, there's the lower-fat items that can take the place of those that are higher in fat, like baked potatoes instead of french fries, or a fruit cup instead of fried eggs. Obvious substitutions like that. And that includes the side items like the butter they give you for your bread or the fat-filled salad dressings—those additions to the meal can easily double the amount of fat the entire meal has."

"It's still a world of choices," Karen said.

"That's exactly right. It'll never be like our fat-reduced, personally designed haven at home, never be like my restaurant, but sensible choices can still be made."

Why aren't there restaurants like yours? Karen thought, before Fowler went on to say, "And with the sugar, that's usually the dessert part of the meal, and there, too, the choices become obvious. Even the choice to just skip the dessert and have only a coffee. And, finally, with the size of the meal, well, the two of us can *share* a meal. Or order one meal and one snack and mix and match that for two. Or ask for a doggy bag for Courage. Or, the one I usually use, *just don't expect to eat it all*. Know in advance that they're going to heap on the food, try to impress you that way, and just eat until you're not hungry, then ask them to take away the rest. *Don't let them sucker you into lead-filled beach-ball territory.*"

Karen was nodding her head.

"But for today," Fowler said, leaning back in his chair, "why don't we do this." He called the waitress over and said, "My daughter and I are ready to order, and if you could just give us a few more minutes after I've ordered, for the lady to think about her choice, I'd appreciate it."

"Sure thing," the waitress answered.

"Okay," Fowler said to her. "My daughter will have the pancakes. I'll have the Spanish omelet, the home-fried potatoes, and — " He faced Karen again and said, "Remember when you ordered bacon at my house, and I said that though it wasn't a food I allowed into my fat-reduced haven, it was still available on The Power of One, because every food can be slotted into at least one of the strategies?"

"I remember that," Karen said.

"Good," Fowler said. Then, turning to the waitress again, he completed his order. "I'll also have a side order of crispy bacon."

The waitress finished writing down the order, then told Fowler she'd come back in five minutes for the last one.

"Thanks," Fowler said. He waited a moment for her to walk away, then said to Karen, "Listen carefully, because this is the best gift The Power of One has to offer."

"Okay..."

Fowler said, "*Strategy number eight. The last strategy of The Power of One—every once in a while, when the urge or circumstance dictates, you can knowingly, and without any sense of guilt, eat foods that don't fit into the guidelines of the other strategies.*" He paused for a moment, letting this last strategy sink in, before he said, "And this isn't just a suggestion or some sort of escape hatch or anything like that. This is a strategy to be followed like all the others. To be assessed and tailored and followed. And there are valid scientific reasons for it." He looked at Janice.

"You tell her," Janice said.

But Fowler shook his head. "You're the scientist in the family." He waited.

Janice, her head slightly bowed and her voice barely above a whisper, said, "This strategy is based on commonly known principles of how the body works. When your focus on all the other strategies reaches a certain level, a level you'll get to quickly, what happens is that without you realizing it, you begin to take in less calories than you used to."

"That's why the weight comes off," Karen said.

"Yes," Janice answered, lifting her eyes a little higher to meet Karen's. "That's why the weight comes off. But after a while the body begins to think that this reduced number of calories is the way it's going to be from now on, so it says to itself, 'Well, if that's the case, if we're only going to have this number of calories from now on, then we'd better *slow down our metabolism to save our fat for times of famine.'* But we don't want that to happen. We don't want our metabolisms to slow down, because that just defeats the purpose of what we're trying to do. So we have to fool the body."

"Fool it?" Karen said.

"Yes. Fool it into believing that we aren't, on the whole, reducing our caloric intake. And we do that by every once in a while eating a larger than usual amount of calories." She turned to Fowler.

Fowler said to Karen, "Remember, we're not talking about pigging out. Just walking away from the other strategies for a meal or two or three, every once in a while. A breakfast here, a lunch there. Dinner. Whatever."

"And that's a strategy?" Karen said. "I mean, going off the strategies is a strategy? It's something I'm supposed to do?"

"That's right. Going off the strategies, every once in a while, when the urge or the circumstance dictates, is one of the strategies. The last strategy. *It's something you're supposed to do. Have to do.* And just like all the other strategies, there's no specific timing to it, no numbers to count, very little to think about."

"And no guilt? You said that, didn't you? No guilt."

Janice laughed, quickly caught it, and dropped her head. Then, lifting her eyes to Karen again, said, nodding toward Fowler, "At the beginning that was his biggest problem too, feeling guilty about going off the other strategies. And he didn't want to do it. Even though he understood the science and explained it to me, he didn't want to do it."

"But I did do it," Fowler said. "Because I wanted to see what would happen. And it works. That blip, that—jolt to the system, keeps the body off guard, keeps it thinking that everything is the way it used to be. This strategy doesn't make you put on weight, because it keeps your metabolism up, and that keeps pushing your weight down."

Fowler smiled at the expression of dubious glee on Karen's face. "And it's this strategy, too, of eating a relatively high-fat meal once in a while, tied to our first strategy of eating as little fat as possible, that keeps our fat levels up to where they should be for our health's sake. Because eliminating any major nutrient, whether it's fat or protein or carbohydrates, is *bad for your health.*"

Janice said to Karen, "This strategy also clearly shows why The Power of One isn't a diet. That it's not something you start and eventually stop. That it is, as my father keeps saying, a way to incrementally, and consistently, over your lifetime, gain health through an understanding of good nutritional practices. Through the understanding of how to defeat those cultural forces that are making fortunes seducing us into buying what they have to offer."

"With this strategy," Fowler said, "though we're fighting a war, and it is a war, The Power of One always remains partnered with the real world. And in the real world there are situations that come up when following the strategies is just not possible. That's when I let this last strategy come into play. When some editor invites me to dinner or when a publisher puts out a spread for an office party, or for any holiday. Or," Fowler said, looking directly into Karen's eyes, "*simply when I get the urge to have something I haven't had in a while,* like bacon. Or, in my case, if it's my sweet tooth that needs to be fed, ice cream."

Karen smiled. She shook her head in wonder.

"So you see," Fowler said again, "leaving the strategies once in a while isn't only one of the strategies, *it's also an important part of the whole process.* First of all, it works on the metabolism, keeps that running at the speed it should. And secondly, it forces The Power of One to fit into the real world, because it says that any food eaten once in a while — even foods that don't fit into the other strategies — are acceptable in this strategy. So that means that in the big picture, the real-life picture, any and every food is okay. *And there are no exceptions to this strategy.* The type of food just doesn't matter."

For a moment no one spoke. Then Karen said, "The Power of One *does fit everyone*, doesn't it? Fits all of us like a second skin. And it's made to wear for the rest of our lives."

"Learn the strategies," Fowler said. "Understand them. Then begin each one slowly, adjusting it to fit you and the particular moment. Then let the strategy, let The Power of One itself, be result-driven. Let your depth of focus depend on the excitement those results create. That'll drive the whole process. And at the same time know that once the knowledge of The Power of One is inside you, the tools to control your nutritional health are in your hands. And know too that you're living in the real world, in real time, with real circumstances and real urges and real walls, and that they're all a part of the whole. All accounted for."

"It has to work," Karen said with certainty.

"Once you have the knowledge," Fowler said, "you can decide to *ignore* that knowledge, pretend you're still blind to the battle going on around you, pretend you don't know the effect the Enemy, the culture, is having on your family's health and your own. But if you do accept the knowledge. If you accept, at any time, any part of any of the strategies, then no, it can't fail. Always remember that you're not attempting something, so you can't fail at it. You're doing it. You're taking a step, then another, then another, toward better health. *And each of those steps is a success in itself, and each success adds to the next, building greater and greater successes.* And if a wall gets in your way, *and it will*, then you take it down when you can, *and continue on.*"

Once again the waitress stepped up to their table. She turned to Karen, but it was Fowler who said to her, "I'd like to add something to my order, if that's alright."

"Sure," the waitress said, lifting her pad. "What'll it be?"

"Water," Fowler said to her. "I forgot to order a glass of water. A tall glass of cold water with a wedge of lemon in it." He grinned at the woman, then added, "You'd better make that three."

CHAPTER

33

Karen sat on the living room couch with Gabe in her arms and waited for Gary to come home. She kept saying to herself, You can do this. You have to do this. You have to find the courage!

Gabe, cranky all afternoon, still wavered between tears and a heavy, toothless pout. Karen lifted him close to her lips and, wishing he could understand, whispered, "No matter what happens, I don't want you to worry, because it's going to be okay."

Just then Gary opened the front door and stepped into the town-house. In a single movement he shucked his jacket onto the hall bench and turned toward the living room.

Karen said, "Gary."

"What?" Gary answered, and walked into the room, took a seat on the easy chair, and reached for the tv remote.

"We have to talk," Karen said.

For an instant Gary looked at her, lips tightly sealed, then turned back to the television and clicked it on.

"We can't go on like this," Karen continued.

In a blunt dismissive tone, Gary said, "I'm hungry."

Karen closed her eyes, slowly shook her head. For the moment Gabe remained quiet.

"Are you deaf?" Gary said. "I just came in. I worked the whole day. I'm hungry."

"No," Karen answered, lifting her eyes to his.

"No? What do you mean, no?"

"I mean we can't go on like this."

Gary stared at her.

"Gary," Karen said, "It doesn't have to be this way, with this much anger. We were good together once. Don't you remember? We fought. But then we made up. Laughed. We were there for each other."

For a long moment, Gary said nothing.

Karen said, "Gary."

"Things change," Gary said.

"But they can change back," Karen quickly replied. "If we try. If we both try. Hard. If we remember how it was. We can do it." She leaned forward. "Please, Gary," she whispered.

Karen watched his jaws tighten, his muscles stiffen. Watched him turn back to the television and say once again, "I'm hungry."

At this, Karen's own expression grew determined. She took a deep breath, stood, and, holding securely to Gabe, said, "Then I've had enough, Gary. I'm a person too. Not your doormat. Not the maid. Not someone who lives here but sleeps on the couch. I won't live this way anymore. I want you out."

"What?"

"I said I want you out!" Karen suddenly screamed. "Get out of this house and get out of my life! I don't want to live with you anymore. Can't you understand that? I'm tired of the insults, of trying to keep you happy, of being a failure just because you say I'm a failure!"

Gabe started to cry. Karen began to rock him, trying to quiet him.

Gary, watching her, said, "If you're finished, I'm still hungry."

"Didn't you hear what I said?"

Gary shrugged his shoulders, the movement slow, filled with disdain, then with an abrupt change of expression he shouted, "The show's over, Karen! You made your splash and you're not going anywhere! If you don't want to sleep on the couch, then don't! I don't care. Is that what you wanted to hear?"

After a long pause, Karen whispered, "Yes." Then, shaking her head, she added, "But it's not enough. I need more than that." She brought her head close to Gabe's. Kissed his tears.

Gary, turning back to the tv, said, "What... more? What do you mean, more?"

"More, Gary. I need more than just permission to sleep in my own bed. I need... respect."

"Then respect yourself," Gary said without looking at her.

Now, for a moment, Karen was silent. Then she said, "I do respect myself. I'm learning how to do that."

"Well good for you."

"And I want you to leave."

"Why do you keep saying that!" Gary shouted, snapping his head toward Karen again. "That's not what you want. You and the kid can't manage on your own. You know that. Not on your salary. Not with the way you are."

"I want you to leave."

Gary turned back to the tv.

Again Karen said, "I want you to leave."

Gary remained silent. Made no movement. Kept his eyes on the television screen.

Karen stepped around to the front of the easy chair. She looked down at Gary and felt, for the first time in her married life, that he was afraid to look at her. Afraid to lift his head, afraid to see what was in her eyes. In a quiet voice she said, "We're finished, Gary. Accept that." And with this she turned from him and stepped to the window, repeating, "Go, Gary. I don't need you anymore."

For a long moment there was no sound between them. Then Gary said, "Karen."

But she didn't turn to him. For an instant she felt guilt, wavered with that, then fear that he'd get violent, storm from the chair and grab her. Then she returned to anger, and let that emotion shunt those other feelings aside, buffer her new-found strength, her growing confidence. She forced herself to keep her back to Gary even when he yelled, "You're going to regret this, Karen. Mark my words!"

She remained steadfast while he stormed to the door and slammed it shut behind him, then watched as he hurried to his car and, with a squeal of tires, drove off.

Now, she knew, she was alone.

She brought her head down to Gabe's, touched his cheek with hers, felt fresh tears rise to just below the surface, and told herself, No! There are a million good reasons to cry. But Gary is not one of them. Not anymore.

She was scared. She admitted that to herself. Take one step, she thought, then another. Remember that each step is a success in itself. Concentrate on that. Only that. She took a deep breath, then whispered to Gabe, "I did it, didn't I? I came up to the wall, and went through it. I went through it. I was scared and I faced it and went through it." She smiled. Felt relief. Felt... hungry.

She went into the kitchen and put Gabe into his seat.

All she'd had to eat today was breakfast with Fowler and Janice, then a burger and fries in the car for lunch. She'd spent the rest of the afternoon thinking about what she was going to do when Gary got home. Building up the courage to go through with it. To either take the steps to make it better. Or end it.

She opened the fridge. There was leftover pizza. Chicken in a bucket. Ice cream in the freezer.

But she wanted none of that.

She smiled. She was staring into the fridge and smiling, just now filling with the excitement and importance of what she'd done. "I did it! I took down my wall!" She shut the fridge door, laughed, then shed a few good tears, knowing that tomorrow she'd begin the formal process of leaving Gary. Tomorrow she'd step from this life into a new one.

The Power of One was in her, she knew. She'd learned the last of the strategies today. The knowledge was there. It could not be erased.

Courage, she thought. Creativity. Tailor the eight strategies to the moment. Take a step, one small step, then another, knowing that each step is a success in itself. Begin a constant, incremental movement toward better health. Toward tomorrow.

She opened the fridge door once again. She took out a lemon, cut a wedge from it, then dropped the wedge into a glass and filled the glass with water.

CHAPTER
34

Fowler, with Gabe in his arms, opened the front door. Gabe squealed when he saw Karen. She reached for him.

Janice, guiding her wheelchair toward them, said, "How did it go?"

Karen smiled. She was wearing a stylish suit and jacket and matching shoes, and in the last seven months had lost twenty-six pounds. The weight loss showed on her face and on her body and in her spirit.

Fowler had told her to go slow and experiment with the strategies. "Make them really yours," he'd said, "not a carbon copy of mine. Work at having The Power of One become invisible in your life."

And she had done so, relishing her steady gain in health and knowing that her steady decline in weight was *permanent.* That every pound lost was not the result of dieting, but of *continuously incorporating small lasting changes into her nutritional lifestyle, her nutritional mind-set.*

She'd had fits and starts, especially during the first few months. She'd accepted them, anticipated they would crop up, and knew too that walls were also going to show themselves. But she had never let herself get caught up in the diet mentality of anxiety and guilt.

She read and reread her notes, finding more in them each time, until The Power of One became firmly planted in her mind, and then gradually, with one small step, and then another, and another, became a part of her life.

Only this morning, when she'd had a coffee with Janice and Fowler before leaving Gabe with them, she likened the eight strategies to friends. "When you first meet someone," she'd said, "it takes time for that person to become a friend, and then a good friend, and then the best of friends. You have to get to know them first, understand them, accept and trust them. And that's the way I approached each of the strategies, anticipating the best, but taking the time I needed."

Now she said to Janice and Fowler, "I got it. I got the loan."

"Yes!" Janice shouted.

"Well, what do you know," Fowler said. "I didn't think they'd be that smart."

"They loved the idea!" Karen said. "The bank manager himself said I could count on him becoming a faithful customer." She laughed. "I can hardly wait to tell Sue and the others in my office. Most of them are already working with The Power of One strategies, and they're getting their families and friends involved too. Even the people who don't need to lose weight are excited about it, about having a way to get a handle on their health. And that's one of the reasons I want this restaurant, so it can become a meeting place for those who want to learn about The Power of One, who want to lose weight without dieting." She shook her head, as though in wonder, then said, "It'll be small, but perfect! And mine! And there'll be no rules broken. No shortcuts taken. Everything I've learned and every ounce of courage and creativity I have will go into it."

"You told him about the menu," Fowler said, "how each item will have the recipe printed too, so your customers can try it for themselves at home? Adapt it to their own strategies?"

"Yes. And he loved that."

"And the takeout counter," Janice said. "That it'll be called the Energy Bank. You told him about that?"

Karen, smiling broadly, nodded.

"What about the name?" Fowler wanted to know.

"With your permission," Karen said, "I'd like to call it The Power of One."

Fowler nodded his head. Karen could see him swallow hard. Then he said, "I would be thrilled for you to use that name. I never imagined anyone else would appreciate it, understand how much significance it has."

"Thank you," Karen whispered. Then, excited again, she said, "The Power of One, a restaurant based on nutritional sanity. And it'll be innovative. I want to give demonstrations on how to find and eliminate fat and sugar, how to work with the other strategies. I'm going to start clubs... Power of One clubs so families and groups of friends can get together, become involved, and help each other take control of their health and weight."

"It's what we've needed for a long time now," Fowler said." Then he turned to Janice. "Looks like this is a day for good news." He stepped closer to her and put a hand on her shoulder.

"I accepted a job offer this morning," Janice told Karen. "They called just after you left."

For a moment Karen had no words, then in a rush she went over to Janice and, with Gabe still in her arms, leaned down and hugged her. "I'm so happy for you."

Janice said, "It's a little scary. But I'm excited. Most of it will be over the internet. But there will be some meetings. I'll have to get on a plane and fly to conferences. I've never even been on a plane before."

Fowler beamed.

Karen said, "The Power of One got you this far, and from here it will take you to wherever you want to go. You, Fowler, me—and the world."

What now?

WHAT NOW?

Okay, you've read *Lose Weight with The Power of One*, met Janice and Fowler, and watched how they led Karen onto the path of nutritional sanity.

Now what do *you* do?

In The Power of One, you saw that the necessary first step to solving your problem is finding the courage to *learn what you need to know to begin your journey.*

Well, you've found that courage, and proven it by reading this book. And by reading this book you've acquired the knowledge. You have in you now the actual *guidelines* you need, the eight strategies to put *your* solution into effect!

And so now is the time to... *relax.* Let the excitement you're feeling at having the solution to your weight problem, flow through you. Savor the moment. Know that The Power of One is now a part of you. Know, without a doubt, that the next step you take, whatever *your* next step is, will be a *small* one. The *smallest, most important step you'll ever take!*

Then you'll take another, and another. Gaining experience and confidence. All the time knowing that what you're doing is changing your nutritional lifestyle, for *life!* Taking these small simple steps, at a pace *you find comfortable*, will bring down your weight and keep it off permanently. Because these changes *are permanent.*

And with every step, The Power of One *will slip deeper into your life*, and soon disappear, the way it did for Fowler.

And like Karen, let your excitement in The Power of One *build*. Use that excitement. Keep it going. Just as Karen had Fowler and Janice, become the nucleus of your own Power of One group. Begin with your children, your family, your friends, then move outward. Let's shout out that there is a way to lose weight easily and permanently. Without dieting! And it's called *Lose Weight with The Power of One!*

A WORD ABOUT EXERCISE

Being a Certified Fitness Trainer, I cannot let you go without at least a short note about exercise.

* Exercise will keep you more focused on The Power of One.

* Exercise will relieve stress.

* Exercise is the magic pill that will first slow your body's aging clock, then reverse it.

* Exercise will change the shape of your body, letting it once again defy gravity.

* Exercise, like The Power of One, will change your life.

Exercise is so vital in my life that I made the conscious decision to not include it in this book. That is because exercise is too important to just tack onto a book about nutrition. It deserves — and I will give it — as full an airing as I did nutrition.

But now that you know a little about me, and my style of conveying new ideas, you can be sure that my book on exercise will be unlike any other you've ever read.

And so I invite you to soon follow Karen, Fowler, and even Janice into the world of fitness. See how they first hit the same wall most of you have, and then gradually discover that exercise, like The Power of One, can be easy, stimulating, and fulfilling. Watch too as their lives, like all of ours, continue to develop.

Stephen Moss

APPENDIX A

Karen, Janice, and Fowler on Spiders, Diets, and Diet Myths

Karen laughed. "What are you doing?"

Fowler, hunched over the coffee table in the living room with his miner's lamp on his head and a magnifying glass in his hand, was staring at a single leaf, placed on a sheet of white paper. "I'm studying a spider," he said. "A little guy called a mite."

"Red spider mite," Janice said, following Karen. Gabe was in her lap, solidly held with one of her small arms, while her other hand rested on her wheelchair's black lever. The baby was freshly changed and fed. "My father likes to see how they eat their way through the leaves," Janice said, looking at Gabe, who was listening intently.

Fowler lifted his head and switched off his lamp. "No diet for this guy."

"And lucky for him," Karen said, taking a seat on the sofa. "Because diets don't work. Isn't that what you always say?"

"That's right," Fowler said, leaning back in his easy chair. "Diets don't work, but they do get you to lose weight."

"What?"

Fowler grinned. "Diets work *for about five minutes*, then the weight gets gained back, plus more."

"I know that's true," Karen answered. "That's what always happened to me before The Power of One. But why is that? I mean, those diets, the fad diets, are so popular. The bookstores are filled with them. Like ***protein diets***. You know the ones. They're all the rage."

Janice laughed.

Fowler said, "Don't even get me started!" He removed the lamp from his head and set it on the table. "Look, Karen, those poor desperate people who get suckered into 'low-carb' or 'high-protein' diets do lose weight initially, even quickly. That's the gimmick. The hook. Only thing is, most of that lost weight is water."

"Water?"

"That's right."

"How can that be?"

"It's like this," Fowler said. "Carbs, as we already know, are our body's preferred fuel—*numero uno*. Potatoes, rice, pasta. Vegetables. Fruits. All of that and more. And so once you stop *adding* carbs to your tank, you quickly use up what's already in there. What happens next is the body goes to plan B and begins to use stored carbs—"

"Glycogen," Janice said. "That's the fancy name for stored carbs."

"Right," Fowler said. "Glycogen. And the body takes that glycogen from the liver and muscles. But the thing is, a lot of water is stored in the body *with* glycogen. In fact *water and glycogen are joined at the hip*, so as you use up those stored carbs, you use up water. A lot of it. And water is heavy, so you lose weight—eight, ten, twelve pounds in a week or two. But is that a real weight loss? Of course not."

"All that's happening is that you're getting dehydrated," Janice said. "Which is dangerous to your health. The weight you really want to lose is body fat, nothing else." Then she said to Fowler, "Tell her the rest."

"The rest is even worse," Fowler said. "Once those *stored carbs* are used up, with all that water, the body has to rely on protein and fatty acids for energy. And because of this, it produces something called ketones. And these, for a whole slew of reasons, are dangerous. But the body, being naturally smart, tries to get rid of the ketones through the liver and kidneys by peeing them out. Unfortunately, this makes you lose even *more water*, causing an even more dangerous situation."

"Those diets work *against* nature," Janice said. "And on top of that, a lot of those low-carb, high-protein diets are also high in saturated fat. They actually tell you to *eat way too much* of that stuff, which can cause a whole other set of serious problems."

Karen shook her head. "It's what you've always said — if it isn't *commonsense,* then it's *nonsense.* "

"Sure is," Fowler said.

"And then, "Janice continued, "There's *food combining*."

Fowler grimaced. "The food combiners have an even more unique gimmick. They say that our digestive system gets sort of *confused* when we eat something like meat and potatoes together. Protein and carbs. And they do so using all these big fancy words — "

"That have no basis in fact or science," Janice added.

"That's right," Fowler said. "But because of that first bit of voodoo, they tell us to eat either one or the other, but never both together. Which, of course, is ridiculous, especially for a meat-and-potatoes kind of guy like me. Or, even stranger, some of them say you have to follow *their plan* of eating certain foods in certain orders, like a fruit twenty minutes before pasta, or some other bit of nonsense."

"Our bodies weren't designed that way," Janice said. "Not even close. They're much more ingenious than that. Our digestive juices, called enzymes, which come from our mouth, stomach, pancreas, liver, and intestine, all *work together*."

"For any kind of food?" Karen asked.

"Any kind and every kind," Fowler said. "Food combining, like protein dieting, is just another gimmick designed to trap well-meaning people into spending their money."

"There's a lot of that out there," Karen said. "***Diet myths***. The average person really doesn't know what to believe... or disbelieve."

"There sure is," Fowler said. Then, shrugging, he added, "Why don't we go through a few of them?" He looked at Janice. "Toss out the ones we laugh at most, and I'll shoot them down." Then he said, "Wait a second," and hurried into the kitchen, coming back moments later with a spatula stuck between the prongs of a fork. He held this at chest height like a machine gun. "Okay, I'm ready, and make it fast, 'cause I'm hot!"

Karen laughed.

"You have to skip meals and starve to lose weight," Janice said quickly.

Fowler raised his "gun" and said loudly, "Crazy! That'll just slow your metabolism, drive you nuts, make you hungry, and at the first wrinkle in your life you'll give up and stuff your face! Next!"

"You can't eat *bad* food, only *good* food."

"Nutso! Food is food. And except for sushi I love it all. Follow the strategies. Next!"

"Carbohydrates like bread, pasta, and rice are fattening, and—"

"Stop there! I love those guys. How dare you lie about them!"

Again Karen laughed.

Janice said, "The key to losing weight is to eliminate fat."

"What! What about my burgers, my fries fix, my Chinese? Forget that nonsense. We need fat, we love fat, and if we'd just *stop swimming in it*, we'd be fine. Next!"

"Liquid diets—"

"Don't even go there! Next!

For a moment Janice paused. Then she said, "Certain foods, like grapefruit, celery, cabbage soup, or vinegar, can burn fat and make you lose weight."

"The only thing that burns fat is your metabolism. Eat enough cabbage and you'll look like one. Next!"

"Eating at night makes you fat."

Karen said, "I think that one—"

Fowler shook his head. "Food is food, eating is eating. Eat too much at any time and you'll get fat. Eat the right amount but only at night, and you'll lose weight. The time you eat makes no difference."

"Okay," Janice said, "here's a good one. You ready?"

"Go for it," Fowler said.

Janice smiled. "A really good diet will get you to lose ten pounds in a week."

Fowler snorted. "I know of a diet that'll let you lose thirty pounds in thirty seconds. It's called the chainsaw diet." Then he raised his spatula and said, "Fast weight loss is only water. The quicker you lose your weight, the sooner you'll gain it back, plus more. The only *permanent weight loss* is weight that's lost through a permanent change in your nutritional life."

"The Power of One," Karen said.

Fowler dipped his head.

"What about me and my slow metabolism?" Karen asked.

Fowler said to Janice, "That's your area."

Janice said, "Having a slow metabolism is a common myth, an easy excuse. The truth is that the difference between a slow and fast metabolism is so minor that it's impossible for that by itself to be a cause of overweight."

"Here's one that I love," Fowler said. "You have to eat according to your blood type." He grinned.

"That makes about as much sense as eating according to the color of your socks!" Janice said, asking next, "What about eating foods according to their glycemic index?"

"What's that?" Karen asked.

Fowler raised his spatula. "Bang! That's where they tell you something as wonderful as a carrot is 'bad' for you. Who do these people think they're fooling?"

Karen sighed. "They're fooling millions."

"There should be a list," Janice said, "of the things to look for when someone tells you about a 'diet.' And if anything on this list sounds familiar, run away fast!"

"Then let's make that list," Fowler said. "And I'd start with that quick weight loss. If they say you'll lose more than a pound or two a week, hightail it out of there."

"And," Janice said, "if they say any food is 'bad' then turn around."

"What about pills?" Karen said. "Or liquids or something like that?"

"Run!" Both Janice and Fowler yelled together.

Karen laughed.

Fowler said, "If they say count calories and keep the number very low, take off! And if they're in it to sell their own food, skeedaddle."

"Skeedaddle?" Janice said.

"Yessiree Ma'am," Fowler said to her. "Karen, the first thing we have to do when we're ready to solve our weight problem is switch on our commonsense, and realize that *losing weight the right way means doing it healthily, and in a manner that will keep it off, for good. For the rest of our lives.*"

"Well, I'm glad to say I'm already doing that," Karen said. "And for me, it's called The Power of One."

APPENDIX B

Karen, Janice and Fowler on Orchids and The Energy Bank

"They're beautiful," Karen said, gently reaching out and touching one of the waxy flowers.

"Beautiful and tough," Fowler said. "Completely deceptive."

"Tough?"

"Oh yes. A plant myth if there ever was one."

"What do you mean?"

"Well, when you say the word *orchid*, most people get a sense of this delicate bloom grown in special greenhouses by the very wealthy. But it's really not like that. Orchids are among the hardiest of plants, growing virtually everywhere, from the tropics to the far north."

"I had no idea," Karen said.

"Just give them a bright window, less water than you'd think, and they'll happily bloom for months each year."

"My favorite is the Cattleya," Janice said, maneuvering her wheelchair over to the long wooden table that sagged beneath the weight of dozens of plants. She'd been working at her blackboard all morning. Now she pointed out an orchid with large white flowers, saying to Karen, "They might be hardy, but there's still a bit of a trick to keeping them looking the way these do." She indicated the space beneath the table.

Karen leaned down and said, "Wow," at the neat rows of potting soils, fertilizers, insecticides, fungicides, pots, stakes, misters, and watering cans.

Fowler grinned. "I like to be prepared for any situation, with my flowers here, and those in the garden."

"Of course you're prepared," Karen said. "You're an expert."

Fowler shook his head. "Experts only become experts over time. With experience. By trying first one thing then another, until the knowledge becomes part of you."

"The Power of One for plants," Karen said.

"That's right," Janice agreed. "Experimenting, getting all his 'strategies' straight. And this," she said, pointing beneath the table, "is like... his energy bank. The freezer."

Fowler smiled.

Karen, though, frowned. "I've started filling my freezer... But between work and Gabe and everything else, it seems to be taking forever. And there are times when I'm really not as prepared as I'd like to be."

"The answer to being prepared," Fowler said, "is to not just focus on your freezer."

"What do you mean?" Karen asked.

"Well," Fowler said, "the freezer is only one of a number of 'tools' you have in your 'energy bank arsenal.' Let me show you."

Janice had turned her chair around and was again staring at her blackboard. Without a word she steered herself to the end of it, erased a few numbers, and stared again.

Fowler grinned, saying, "Well, we lost Janice." Then he motioned Karen to the kitchen. "You already know what's in my freezer, so I don't have to show you that. And actually, for a moment, let's just pretend I don't even have a freezer—at least not one that's filled with precooked food."

"Okay," Karen said.

"Now then, I need a quick snack, a lunch, or even an evening meal. So what do I do?"

"You go to the fridge," Karen began.

"Right. Most people stare inside, and let their eyes glaze over. But in my case, I'm always sure I'll find something appealing, and that fits the Power of One strategies, because the fridge has become one of my weapons." Opening the fridge door, and pointing to the deli counter, he asked Karen, "What do you see?"

"I see two well-stocked fridges. With lots of plastic containers."

"That's another major tool. Containers," Fowler said, reaching for one. He opened it and showed it to Karen. "Tuna salad. Delicious. I made it yesterday, in about two minutes, but instead of using only one can, which is about as much as I can eat at a time, I used three." As he closed the container, he said, "Most of it will gone by tonight, because I'll keep nibbling on it before dinner." He touched another container. "So will the pasta, because that's what Janice is planning on having.

"There's also cooked veggies and salad in a bag, and without even looking I'm sure there's at least one or two other leftovers sitting there, because what's better than leftovers?" Fowler said. "Even if I don't make enough of whatever I'm cooking to pack into the freezer, I'll still always make enough so there's something left over for at least one more snack or meal. And it could be later on, or the next day, or even the day after that."

"Mix-and-match leftovers," Karen said.

"And some of the best meals going," Fowler added. He reached to the back of the fridge and brought out a bowl of hard-boiled eggs. "How's this for a quick snack? Peel off the shells, give the yolk to Courage, break the whites into a small bowl, add salt and pepper, toss in a tomato or bit of onion or anything else you like, and *voila*. Or keep one yolk, and mash up four eggs with fat-reduced mayo and Dijon mustard, and—yum—egg salad."

"And let's not forget everyone's favorite," Karen said. "The sandwich."

Fowler nodded. "Anyone of probably a dozen different low-fat sandwiches can be made with what's in my fridge right at this moment. Make a sandwich on whole wheat or multigrain or a great ethnic bread, and eat half. And save the other half for later.

"Or," he continued, "for a fast snack there's also salmon, or fat-reduced soup from a can, or fat-free pretzels, or chicken hotdogs or Janice's favorite snack of all, a fruit.

"Just like with my flowers, I've become an expert on being prepared with food, mine and Janice's. Our comfort foods. By letting my experience, and experiments, add up. Add to my growing expertise of what Janice and I like, what's simple, and what can stay in the fridge a day or two, or in the cupboard for weeks and months." He smiled. "We always have to eat. There's no getting around that. So, every time I do eat, I let it *work for me*, add to my store of tricks."

"I get it," Karen said. "Being 'prepared' doesn't have to be a big deal. I mean, I'm going to fill my freezer. I'm looking forward to it. But until that's happened— "

"Not just until, but even when your freezer is filled," Fowler said, "there's still a whole arsenal of tasty snacks and meals you can have at a moment's notice."

Karen shook her head. "Every time I think that there's something about The Power of One I have to worry about, I find out it's not true."

"Take your time," Fowler said. "Relax and enjoy the process, and become the expert for *your* family's food. Your core meals and comfort foods. Very quickly, it'll all come to you without a second thought."

APPENDIX C

Karen, Janice and Fowler on Stress

"Gabe was crying most of the night, poor thing," Karen said, placing the sleeping baby onto Fowler's spare bed. "Then at seven this morning Gary called to say he won't be able to make his payment this month, and then when I had Gabe in the car to bring him here, the car wouldn't start. So now I'm waiting for a call from the garage to find out what the problem is." She stood, looked at Janice, and said, "What I need now is a friend, a special friend."

"I'm a friend."

Karen tilted her head. "You know what I mean. The kind of friend I need now is gooey and full of fat and sugar and calories." She feigned a scowl.

Janice motioned her to the kitchen. They could hear a frustrated-sounding Fowler on the phone.

"I'm not happy about it," Karen said, taking a seat at the table. "But I'll admit it. I have a... a..."

"A craving," Janice said. "Why aren't you happy about it?"

"Because it means I'll be bad, taking a step backward for no good reason. And it's going to make me fat, when I'm doing so well."

Janice shook her head. "All you're doing is being human. For most of us the need to use food as comfort once in a while is virtually impossible to fight. It's biological. Emotional. And never debatable. But that's all it is. It isn't bad or good, and it isn't taking a step backward. It just is."

"And it's not going to make you fat," Fowler said, stepping into the kitchen. He walked straight to the freezer, adding, "That was my new editor. He wants an article on carnivorous plants—by the end of the week!" He opened the freezer door with his back to Karen and Janice, blocking their view of what he was doing.

Karen, facing Janice again, said, "What I'm feeling right now is a craving alright. A strong one. But why does it happen?"

Janice shrugged. "There are so many potential causes for why we feel that way about food. If you studied ten different people, you'd come out with fifteen different reasons."

Karen laughed.

"But," Janice continued, "the more important question is what do we *do* about it."

Fowler stepped up to the table with two small bowls of ice cream sprinkled with pecans and doused in chocolate sauce. "Will this cover that craving?" he asked, taking a seat and handing Karen one of the bowls and a spoon.

"Oh my God," Karen said. "Will it ever! You must have read my mind." Then she looked at Janice, as though asking permission.

"Eat," Janice said. "I can bet you my father will devour his in two seconds."

Fowler, working quickly on his ice cream, said, "Karen, does it really matter why there are times when our brains tell our bodies that we need this stuff... now! Or for me it could be a piece of cake or a chocolate bar..."

"Or," Janice said, "an ordered-in, dripping-in-fat pizza, when he's got one of his own delicious low-fat pizzas just waiting to be eaten."

Fowler laughed. "It makes no sense to try to make sense of it. Just accept that this happens, and control it."

"But I thought you said—" Karen began.

"By control," Janice said, "he means keep the portion small."

"Keep the portion as small as possible," Fowler said. "Don't make it a daily habit. Practice putting it off, if you can. But above all, *don't feel guilty*. And don't think it's going to make you fat, because a reasonable amount of anything, every once in a while, is never the problem. It's only eating too much too often that's a problem."

"So what you're saying," Karen said, "is tell myself that there are times — days, mornings like this one — when I don't have to be superwoman. When I can indulge, soothe my frustrations, and feel okay about it."

"Exactly," Fowler said, finishing off the last of his ice cream. "Feel good about it, and feel even better if you don't go for seconds. But if you do, then look yourself in the mirror and say, I deserve this, because it's been one of those days. And let's hope I don't have another like this for a long time. Then blow yourself a kiss, and indulge."

QUICK VERSION
OF THE POWER OF ONE

STRATEGY ONE

Reduce the amount of fat in your daily life to as low as possible

This goes to the heart of our fat-filled culture — getting rid of all the excess fat we're given at every turn. We're swimming in fat, and that's making us fat. The idea is to get rid of it where we can, know that this has absolutely nothing to do with any low-fat diet, and then move on with our lives. Because we all need some fat to be healthy. Here are some tips that will do the job:

- Use fat-reduced items to directly replace their high-fat equivalents, especially dairy products.

- Reduce the number of egg yolks you use.

- Choose lean cuts of meats and poultry, and cut off any visible fat. Remove the skin from poultry.

- Use nonstick spray in nonstick pans when cooking.

- Try defatting ground beef.

- With restaurant meals, reduce or eliminate the "side dish" fats, such as salad dressing, butter, or mayo.

STRATEGY TWO

Eat breakfast

Breakfast is the meal that gets your engine running, letting you begin burning enough calories so you can start your day losing weight. Eating breakfast also keeps you from "starving" by mid-morning and then grabbing anything you can. It should follow the concepts of the other strategies

STRATEGY THREE

Reduce the amount of sugar in your daily life to as low as possible

This one is a lot easier than most people think.

• Reduce your portion sizes of dessert, or share when possible.

• Choose a fruit instead of a pastry.

• Substitute a no-calorie sweetener instead of sugar.

• Drink diet sodas, or, better yet, switch to water.

Most important, do what you can and move on. Play the Power of One game of being more focused today than yesterday, and never beat yourself up over anything. Just get on with life!

STRATEGY FOUR

Do not bring any factory-made snacks or meals, or refined flour products into your home — use foods that are as close to natural as possible

Factory-made foods and snacks are the same as fast food, filled with too much fat and sugar and things no one can pronounce. And refined flour products like white bread have no nutritional value. *As much as possible* we should make our "at-home meals" from whole, fresh foods. It's easy, quicker than you think, puts control of your family's nutrition into your hands, where it should be — and it's exciting to begin to gain health and lose weight.

STRATEGY FIVE

Drink water

Water is our body's most important nutrient. Start drinking it early in the day. Keep a bottle of water with you. Keep another in your car. Ask for water in restaurants. Experiment with it by adding lemon or lime. Let drinking water become second nature.

STRATEGY SIX

Stop eating when you are approaching feeling full but have not yet swallowed the lead-filled beach ball

This one takes work because our bodies tell us when to start eating but not when to stop. In fact, our genetics, always worried about that fictional famine, don't want us to stop eating until all the food in front of us is gone.

Here's how to put this strategy into effect:

• Work with your head, your courage, and the feeling in your stomach. While eating, keep checking how close you are to feeling "not hungry" and how close you are to feeling "stuffed." Know there is a place somewhere between these two feelings that is perfect. And with practice, you'll begin to recognize it.

• Work at using your experience to know just how much to put into your plate, so that you can finish it all and still not enter the "stuffed" zone.

• Keep temptation away. Work at creating a situation where it's easy to say, "That was good. I'm not hungry anymore. I know I can still shove a lot more food down, but I don't have it in front of me — so I won't.

• Practice walking away from what's left in your plate and see how quickly the feeling of needing to eat more disappears. Because it's not a true feeling.

• Let the knowledge of how much is enough become second nature, a habit. Let it become an invisible part of your life.

STRATEGY SEVEN

Eat often

Our bodies were not designed to survive on just three meals a day. Breakfast, lunch, and dinner is a rule our society came up with.

- A good rule of thumb is to eat five or six times a day. Every two or two and a half or three hours. Whatever is convenient.

- Eat just the right amount and the right kind of food to get you to the next meal or snack. Go from mildly hungry, to not hungry, to mildly hungry again, as often as you need to.

STRATEGY EIGHT

Every once in a while, when the urge or circumstance dictates, forget about the other strategies

This is not just a suggestion or some sort of escape hatch. This is a strategy to be followed like all the others. We must do this to fool our bodies into believing that we aren't, on the whole, reducing our caloric intake, so that it won't slow our metabolism.

- This does not mean stuffing ourselves—just walking away from the other strategies for a meal or two every once in a while. Breakfast, lunch, or dinner. When the circumstance or the urge occurs. We also use this strategy of eating a higher-fat-than-usual meal or snack, and adding it to our first low-fat strategy, so that our fat levels are where they should be for a healthy body and mind.

STRATEGIES OF THE POWER OF ONE

1. Reduce the amount of fat in your daily life to as low as possible.

2. Eat breakfast.

3. Reduce the amount of sugar in your daily life to as low as possible.

4. Do not bring any factory made snacks, meals or refined flour products into your home. Use foods that are as close to natural as possible.

5. Drink water.

6. Stop eating when you are approaching feeling full, but have not yet swallowed the lead-filled beach ball.

7. Eat often.

8. Every once in a while, when the urge or circumstance dictates, forget about the other strategies.

**These strategies are all in a guilt-free zone!
Nowhere in your life should you ever let yourself
fall into the "diet mentality" trap!**

Stephen Moss is a novelist,
Certified Fitness Trainer, Specialist
in Weight Management, and a
Lifestyle and Weight Management
Consultant. He and his wife
Natalia live in Montreal, Canada.